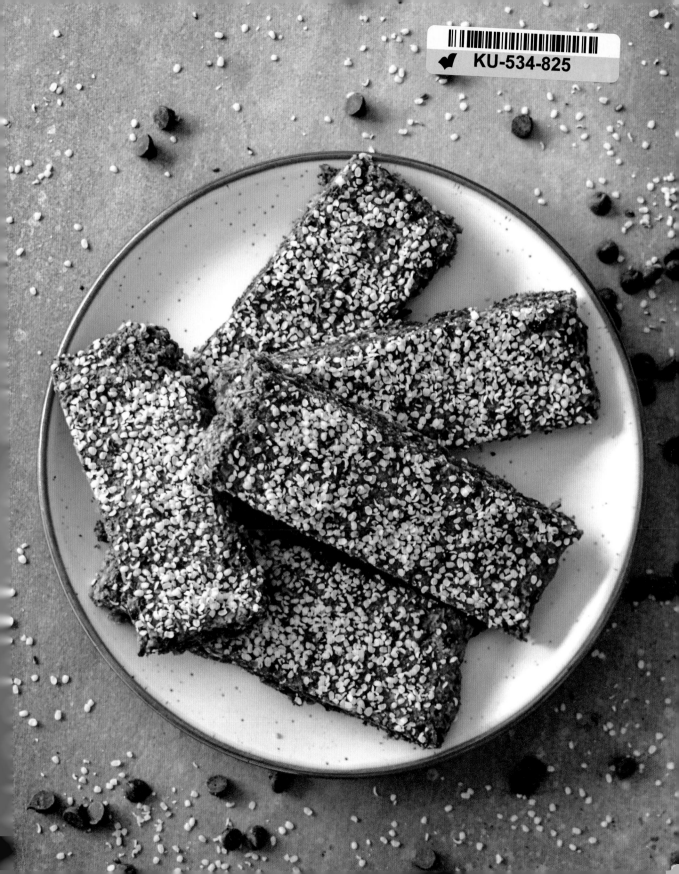

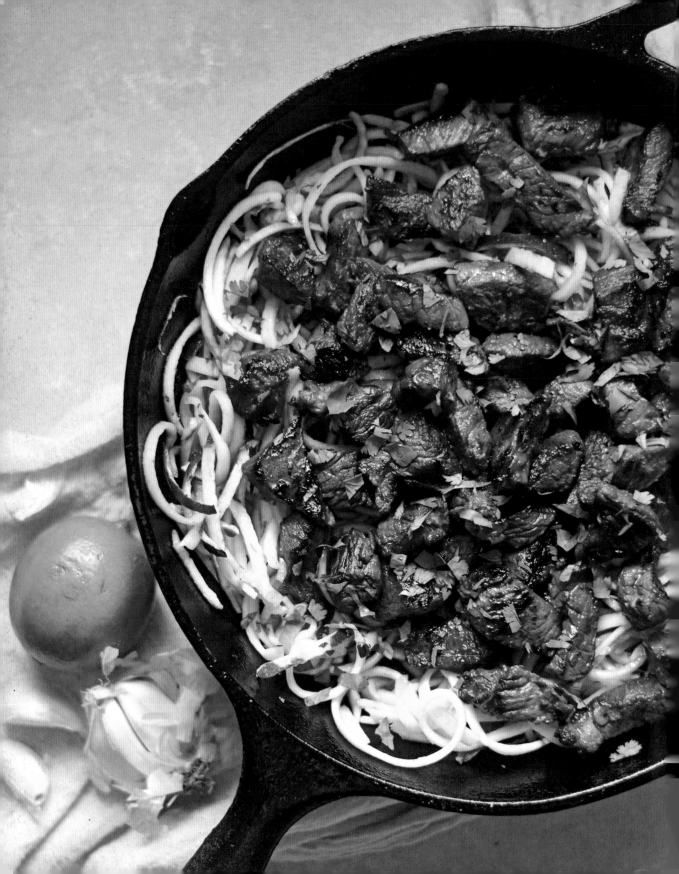

KETO DIET
COOKBOOK

Also by Dr. Josh Axe

Keto Diet

Eat Dirt

KETO DIET
COOKBOOK

**125 Delicious Recipes to Lose Weight,
Balance Hormones, Boost Brain Health,
and Reverse Disease**

Dr. Josh Axe

First published in the United States in 2019 by Little, Brown Spark,
Hachette Book Group

Little Brown Spark is an imprint of Little, Brown and Company, a division of
Hachette Book Group, Inc. 1290 Avenue of the Americas, New York, NY 10104

This edition published in Great Britain in 2019 by Orion Spring
an imprint of The Orion Publishing Group Ltd

Carmelite House, 50 Victoria Embankment London EC4Y 0DZ

An Hachette UK Company

1 3 5 7 9 10 8 6 4 2

A CIP catalogue record for this book is available from the British Library.

ISBN (Trade paperback) 9781409196853

ISBN (eBook) 9781409196860

Cover and print book design by Gary Tooth / Empire Design Studio

Printed in Italy

www.orionbooks.co.uk

Every effort has been made to ensure that the information in the book is
accurate. The information in this book may not be applicable in each
individual case so it is advised that professional medical advice is obtained
for specific health matters and before changing any medication or dosage.
Neither the publisher nor author accepts any legal responsibility for any
personal injury or other damage or loss arising from the use of the
information in this book. In addition if you are concerned about your diet
or exercise regime and wish to change them, you should consult a health
practitioner first.

The publisher is not responsible for websites (or their content) that are not
owned by the publisher.

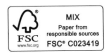

This book is dedicated to my best friend,
my wife, and the love of my life,
Chelsea Axe, and to my father God, for
giving me the platform and favor to
create this book.

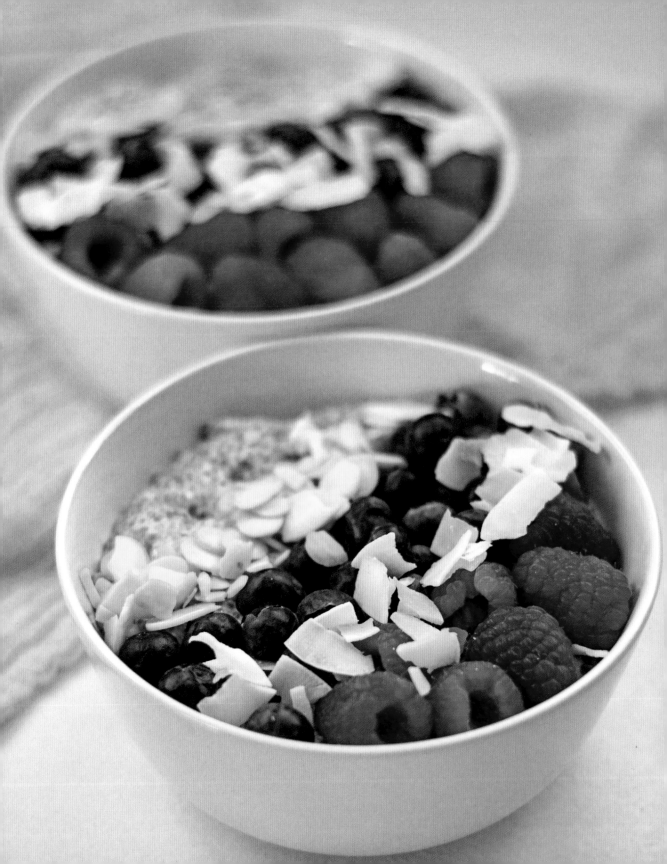

Contents

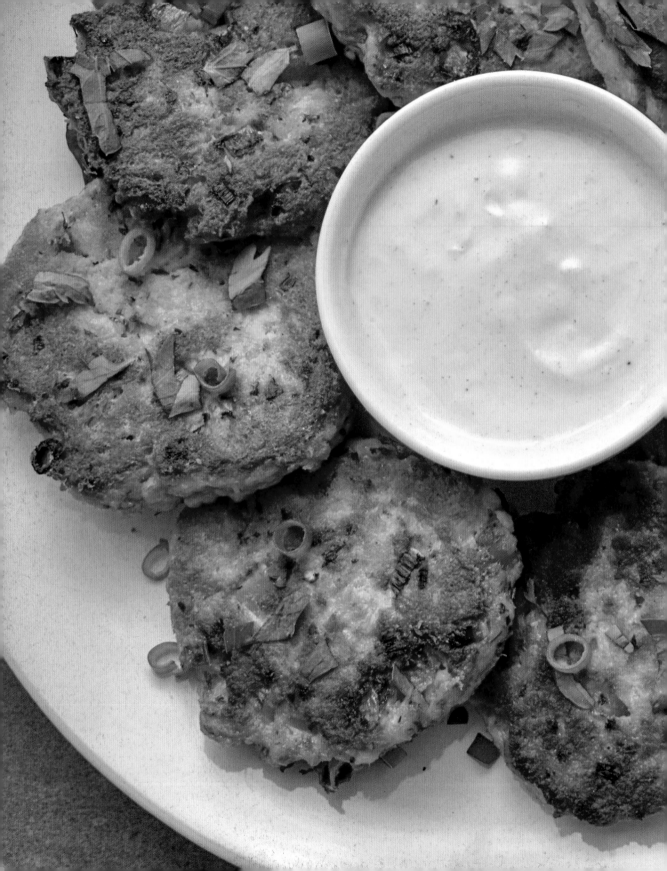

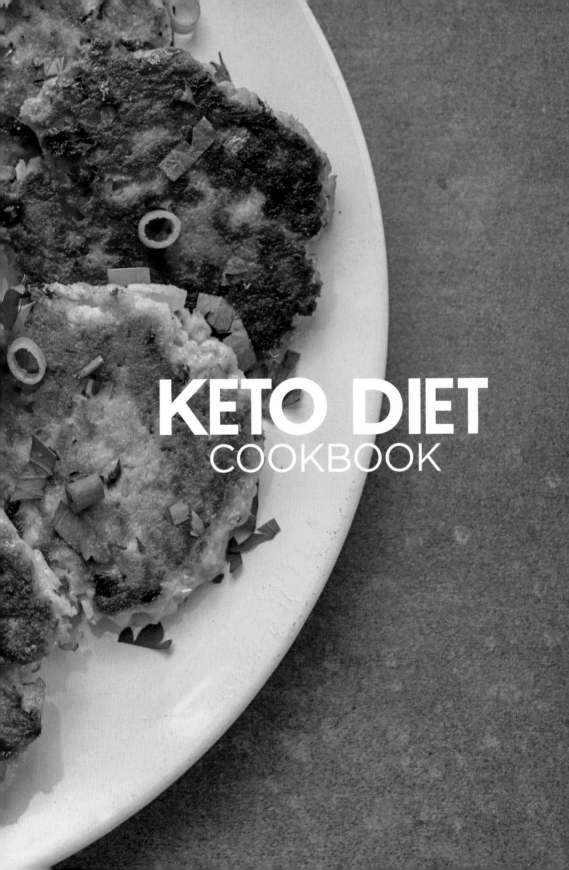

KETO DIET
COOKBOOK

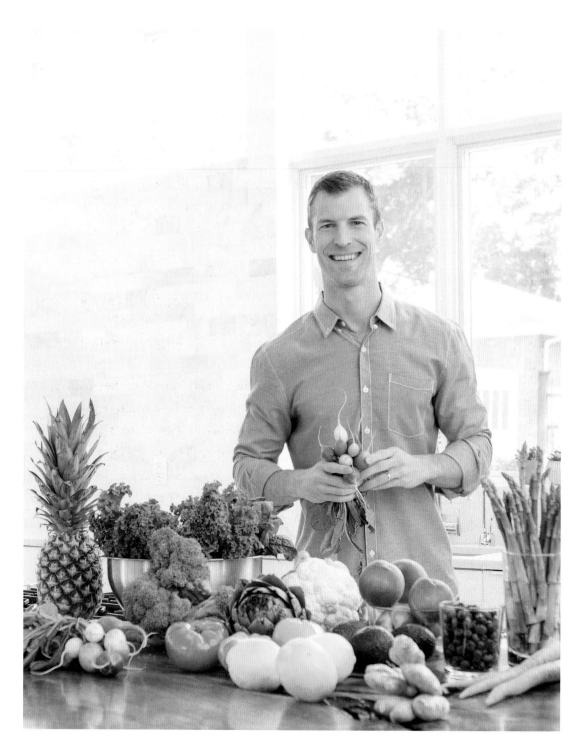

Introduction

If, like so many other people, you haven't had success following diets that require making bland or tasteless recipes, counting calories, limiting yourself to small portion sizes, or cooking with unusual ingredients, then the keto diet may be the game changer you've been looking for. No more going hungry, fighting cravings, cooking flavorless foods, or avoiding some of your favorite foods that actually fill you up and leave you satisfied, like quality oils, real butter, nuts, and more.

Those who have been successful on the keto diet are a testament to just how transformative a clean keto diet and lifestyle can be. Tens of thousands of people have experienced significant improvements in their health by embracing a high-fat, very low-carb lifestyle—whether it's for just a few months or on-and-off for years, depending on their goals.

No other diet is capable of actually shifting your body's source of fuel from carbohydrates to primarily fats. This is why, for many people, virtually no other diet can be credited with such dramatic changes in their physical and mental health. We're talking about changes like a boost in focus, endurance capacity, muscle power, metabolic health, and weight management.

Here's the thing about recipes that are keto-compliant: There's a right way and a wrong way to do it. While it's true that the macronutrient components of the two types of eating plans—a "dirty" keto diet and a "clean" keto diet— may be very similar, the foods that are emphasized differ dramatically. You may be able to stay in ketosis while eating mostly bacon, burgers, and fried cheese, but do you really think this will leave you feeling your best or move you closer to your goals?

If you want to experience a boost in your heart health, cognitive function, physical performance, and mood by following the keto diet, you need to supply your body with the essential vitamins, minerals, fiber, and macronutrients that it needs to thrive. In order not only to lose weight (if this is one of your goals), but also protect yourself from disease and enhance your quality of life, it's critical to cook with nutrient-dense foods. These include healthy fats such as avocado, coconut oil, olive oil, and salmon, and also a variety of vegetables, herbs, broths, and quality proteins. These are the types of healing foods you'll find in the recipes throughout this book.

Whether you're ready to commit 100 percent to the keto diet and eager to jump right into ketosis, or you're simply looking for inspiration when it comes to preparing more nutrient-dense, high-fat, low-carb meals at home, I hope this becomes your go-to cookbook for delicious, health-promoting recipes. I'm confident that with help from the grocery store and your kitchen, you'll find these keto recipes satisfying, simple to make, and worth serving regularly at your table.

Wishing you many blessings,

Dr. Josh Axe

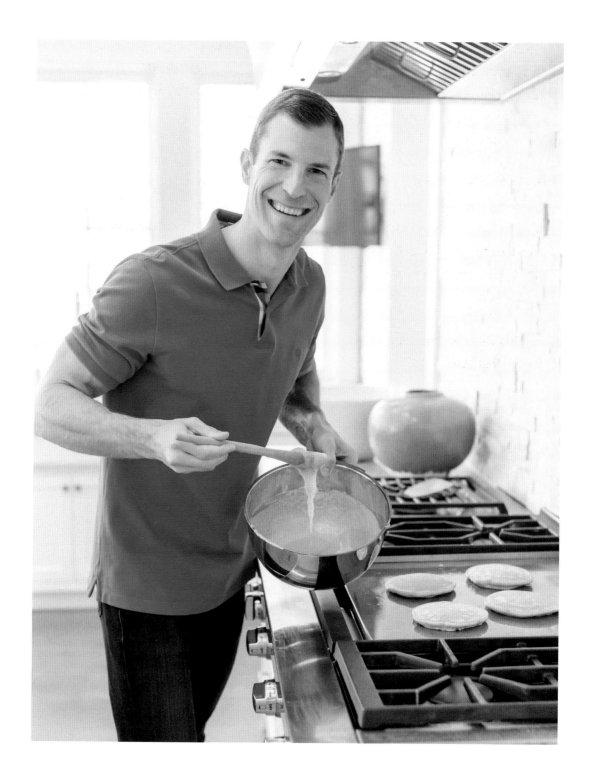

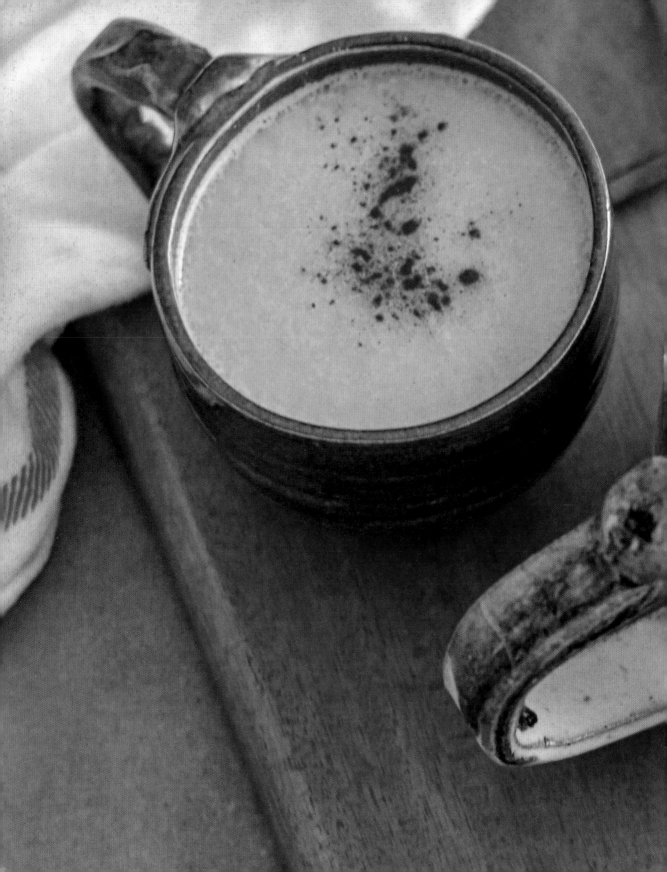

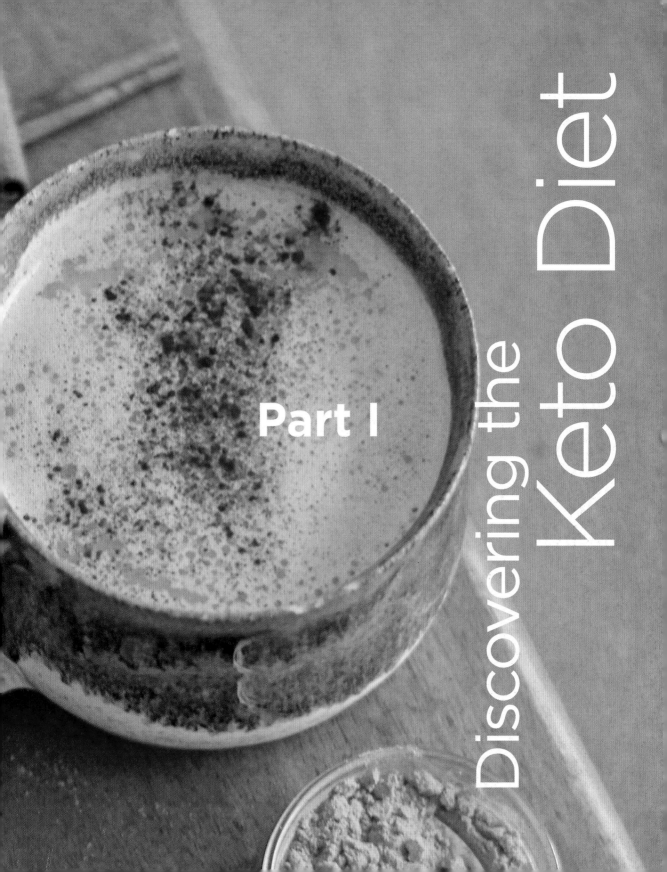

Part I

Discovering the Keto Diet

What Is the Keto Diet?

The ketogenic (or "keto") diet is a high-fat, very low-carb diet that has been used by doctors since the 1920s. Doctors first developed the keto diet to help control seizures among patients with epilepsy.

The purpose of the keto diet is to put your body into a metabolic state called nutritional ketosis, in which you burn fat for energy, rather than glucose from carbohydrates. Ketosis is characterized by raised levels of ketone bodies in the body tissues, which is typically the by-product of eating a diet that is very low in carbohydrates.

Most mammals, including humans, have the ability to use fat for fuel during times of famine, low energy intake, and when carbs are scarce. Our bodies store glucose and reserved glycogen in order to make sure we don't run out of energy, but if no carbs are coming in, these will eventually run out. After several days on a very low-carb diet, our bodies start producing compounds called ketone bodies (or ketones) from our own stored body fat, as well as from fats in our diet, as an alternative fuel source.

Recognizing the Signs of Ketosis

While in nutritional ketosis, ketone bodies provide your brain, muscles, and organs with a steady source of energy. Your body basically operates as a "fat burner" instead of a "carbohydrate burner." Once you become "fat adapted" (i.e., your body can use fat rather than carbs for energy), you should experience not only weight loss but also mental clarity, appetite suppression, improved digestion, and more consistent energy throughout the day.

Here are five signs that you're likely in ketosis:
- **Weight loss:** Many people will notice weight loss quickly due to losing a combination of water weight (from cutting carbs), excess body fat that's being burned, and by reducing inflammation.

- **Reduced hunger levels/appetite:** Ketones are naturally appetite-suppressing, which means it's easier to control calorie intake and to go longer periods of time without eating (i.e., it's easier to practice intermittent fasting if you choose to try this).

- **Stabilized energy:** When your body is in ketosis, you'll experience fewer ups and downs in terms of energy and cravings, since your blood sugar will be steadier.

- **Decreased sluggishness and brain-fog:** Your energy won't only stabilize, but will also show improved endurance and stamina. You can also expect greater mental clarity and sharpness.

AVOIDING KETOSIS OBSTACLES

Below are some habits that can either prevent you from getting into ketosis, pull you out of ketosis, or just leave you feeling run-down even if you are, in fact, in ketosis.

- **Not consuming the right macronutrient ratio:** To enter ketosis, you must consume the ideal macronutrient ratio (see "Your Macronutrient Ratio on the Keto Diet" on page 22). Also, tracking your macronutrient intake is vital to ensuring success on the ketogenic diet, so consider keeping a food journal or using an app for help.

- **Not eating enough fat/calories in general:** This will make it hard to produce enough ketones and lead to symptoms such as fatigue.

- **Eating too much protein:** The keto diet isn't a high-protein diet; it's a moderate protein, high-fat diet (because excess protein can be turned into glucose).

- **Eating processed fats and foods low in nutrients:** Eating these foods can throw off your hunger signals and provide sneaky carbs. Avoid foods with poor quality oils, processed meats, high-sodium foods, fried foods, and fast foods. While you do still need some carbs in your diet, it's best to select high-fiber, nutrient-rich options to keep carb consumption to a minimum.

- **Not eating vegetables:** Eating nutrient-rich vegetables is crucial for getting enough fiber, vitamins, minerals, and antioxidants.

Keep in mind that factors like sleep deprivation, physical inactivity, and even stress can actually hold you back from reaching your keto diet weight loss goals.

Ideally, you want to focus on staying in ketosis while also making holistic and healthy changes to your lifestyle. This combination can help with goals like weight loss or blood sugar management, and will leave you feeling great overall.

- **Less bloating and gas:** This results from cutting out sugar, processed foods, and refined grains from your diet, the primary culprits of gastrointestinal discomfort.

Ketones are a by-product of fatty acid breakdown, and testing your blood, breath, or urine for ketones can be a useful indication of whether or not your body has reached ketosis. If you want to know for sure that you're officially in ketosis, there are several ways to test ketone levels: urine strips (the easiest and most popular method), blood tests, or breathalyzer tests. Keto strips are available at most pharmacies near the diabetic supplies.

The Benefits of Entering Ketosis

By following the keto diet and entering a state of ketosis, you can reap the many benefits of turning your body into a fat-burning machine. Here are the top health benefits of the keto diet.

1. Supports metabolism

When it comes to helping you reach and maintain a healthy weight, the keto diet has a number of unique anti-obesity and disease-modifying effects. The keto diet is unlike any other diet because it forces your body to use fat, from both your diet and your stored adipose tissue, for energy rather than glucose (sugar).

There's evidence that a non–calorie-restricted keto diet (in which you eat to the point of feeling satisfied) may be more effective at helping with weight maintenance compared to a very low-calorie diet. That's because the keto diet can help you hold onto lean muscle mass if you also engage in strength-training exercises, and it doesn't cause your metabolic rate to slow down like many other low-calorie "crash diets" do.

Based on our research findings, people who are overweight and obese can expect the keto diet to significantly reduce body weight and body mass index (BMI), lead to improved appetite control, and also improve their lipid profile and blood glucose levels without causing any significant negative side effects. Although the keto diet alone can definitely lead to weight loss, the effects are even more impressive when it works in tandem with exercise. A keto diet plus exercise can lead to an improvement in fat oxidation, more desirable body composition, and a decrease of RER (respiratory exchange ratio, which shows the muscle's oxidative capacity to get energy), all without significantly reducing your resting metabolic rate.

2. Fights food cravings

One mechanism of the keto diet that leads to weight loss is by reducing your appetite and promoting satiety (the feeling of fullness). This is attributed to a higher intake of filling foods that provide protein and fats that take longer to burn than carbohydrates, and due to the effects that ketones have on appetite-controlling hormones, including ghrelin. Even during a period of weight loss, the keto diet does not typically increase circulating ghrelin levels, and this is a good thing because ghrelin is a hormone that makes people feel hungry.

Many people find that they can control calorie intake more easily and quit snacking on empty-calorie junk foods between meals while in ketosis without feeling deprived. Additionally, because hunger is kept under control thanks to ketones, many people find they can be successful with intermittent fasting if they choose to do this.

3. Balances blood sugar levels

Very low-carbohydrate, high-fat diets are safe and effective when it comes to reducing blood sugar fluctuations in diabetic and pre-diabetic adults. Following a very low-carb diet causes your body to release less insulin, which is an energy-storing hormone that is released into the bloodstream when you consume sugar and carbohydrates.

Because the keto diet prevents excessive release of insulin, it helps to balance blood glucose levels, leading to fewer spikes and dips in blood sugar, which can eventually contribute to metabolic disease. Normalizing blood glucose levels via the keto diet can be useful for reversing "insulin resistance," which is the underlying problem contributing to type 2 diabetes.

4. Promotes heart health

Despite the fact that the keto diet is high in fat—including saturated fat, which is often demonized by health authorities—it can actually have protective effects when it comes to cardiovascular function. This depends on the quality of your food choices, which is why not all fats are created equal, and eating a "clean" keto diet is so important.

The keto diet has been shown to help lower LDL ("bad cholesterol"), to lower triglycerides, and to raise HDL ("good cholesterol"), plus it can help to lower blood pressure and decrease obesity and metabolic syndrome, all of

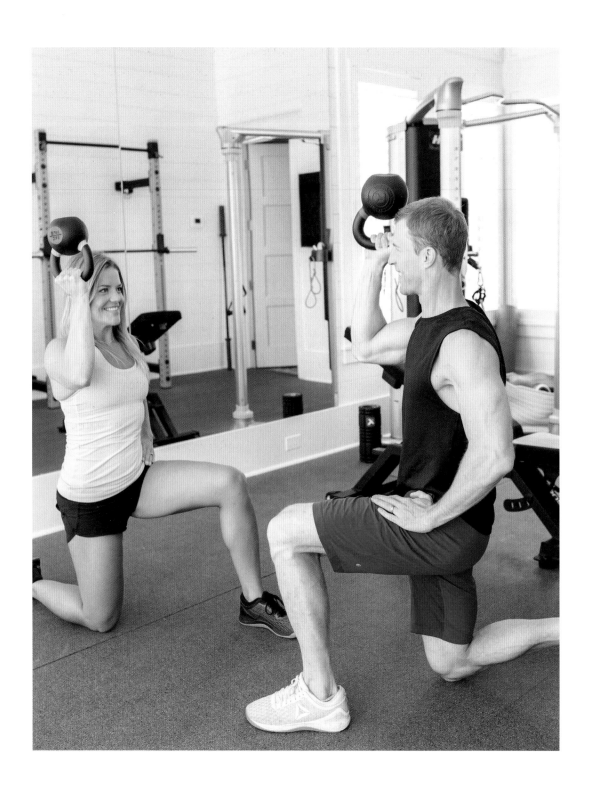

which are linked to heart-related problems. Some studies have found that adults who follow a keto diet tend to achieve better long-term body weight and cardiovascular risk factor management when compared with adults assigned to conventional low-fat diets.

5. Regulates healthy inflammation response

When fat replaces glucose as the body's primary energy source, the body produces three types of ketone bodies (or ketones): acetoacetate, ß-hydroxy-butyrate, and acetone, which studies show have anti-inflammatory effects and protect against cellular injury.

The high fatty acid load of the ketogenic diet seems to activate the body's natural anti-inflammatory mechanisms and improves mitochondrial energy homeostasis, or the way our cells produce and use energy.

Another way in which ketosis fights inflammation is by fatty acids stimulating production of peroxisome proliferator-activated receptor alpha (PPARa), a protein that regulates the expression of certain genes and produces a potent anti-inflammatory response. Ketones also seem to help fight oxidative damage from free radicals and an unhealthy lifestyle. Finally, a clean keto diet can be anti-inflammatory because it includes lots of healing foods like olive oil, nuts, fish, and fresh vegetables, while also eliminating problematic foods with added sugar, refined grains, synthetic additives, and processed oils that all spike inflammation.

6. Keeps hormones balanced

The ketogenic diet has safe and therapeutic effects in both children and adults, especially when it comes to regulating functions of the endocrine, immune, and central nervous systems. In fact, the good, healthy fats that make up 75 percent of the standard keto diet are the same fats that serve as the building blocks for hormones such as estrogen, progesterone, and testosterone. As a result, consuming these fats actually helps support hormone production and balance.

7. Aids brain health

Remember when I mentioned that the keto diet was originally developed to help control epileptic seizures? Studies from the 1920s have shown that the keto diet has a strong neuroprotective effect, mostly due to its ability to reduce inflammation in the brain and normalize insulin levels. The diet has been used clinically for more than 90 years in the treatment of epilepsy and a number of difficult-to-treat neurological disorders. Today research continues to show that ketosis has a number of positive effects on the brain, such as improving the way that the mitochondria in our cells work to produce energy.

There is also evidence that the keto diet offers protection against a broad range of neurodegenerative disorders, including Alzheimer's disease, Parkinson's disease, traumatic brain injury, and stroke. More recently, the diet has also been used to help manage multiple sclerosis (MS), amyotrophic lateral sclerosis (ALS, or Lou Gehrig's disease), Huntington's disease, brain cancer, schizophrenia, autism, and recurring headaches.

Some of the mechanisms by which the keto diet supports cognitive health include providing the brain with sustainable energy in the form of ketones, preventing insulin resistance, balancing blood sugar levels, enhancing cellular metabolic and mitochondrial functions, and protecting cells and neurons in the brain from oxidative stress and damage. While there's still more to learn about these complex mechanisms that lead to neuroprotection, they seem to be tied to enhanced neuronal energy reserves, improved ability of neurons to resist metabolic challenges, and enhanced antioxidant and anti-inflammatory effects in the brain during ketosis.

8. Boosts mental focus

The brain, which normally relies on glucose for energy, can switch to using ketone bodies during periods of glucose restriction, fasting, or starvation. Being in the metabolic state of nutritional ketosis means that your energy-guzzling brain is using fat as fuel, which is a steady, slow-burning energy compared to glucose from carbohydrates, which tends to spike after consumption and quickly dip. In addition to lowering your risk for cognitive disorders, a clean keto diet is also capable of improving high-level cognitive functions and mental performance, such as by enhancing focus, attention, memory, and potentially problem-solving and learning capacity.

If you normally experience brain-fog or an "afternoon slump," you can expect to feel more clearheaded while in ketosis. An added benefit is that you won't need to rely on caffeine and sugar to get you through your day.

9. Encourages uplifted mood

You can thank the steady supply of ketones that your brain receives when you're in ketosis for keeping you feeling levelheaded and energized. Normally, when you're burning glucose for energy, your blood sugar will tend to surge right after eating, then plummet shortly after, especially if you consume lots of processed carbs and sugar. This cycle negatively affects your moods, concentration, and energy. On the other hand, while you're in ketosis, energy will be largely derived from the utilization of your own body fat and from the fat you consume from your diet, which has a slower and steadier release to keep you thriving.

Other ways that the keto diet can protect against mood-related problems, such as the symptoms of depression and anxiety, are by reducing inflammation and helping to balance the release of insulin, a hormone that affects many other hormones in the body that regulate your mood, including cortisol, melatonin, estrogen, and testosterone.

A healthy keto diet can also support gut health, and we know that inflammation inside your gut can affect the release of neurotransmitters like serotonin and dopamine that are needed to keep your mood up. This is one reason why the keto diet may be therapeutic for people experiencing mood swings that are tied to leaky gut or overgrowth of unhealthy bacteria in the gastrointestinal tract derived from a high-sugar diet, chronic stress, or exhaustion.

10. Increases energy levels

Staying in ketosis helps to stabilize blood sugar by turning the body into a fat-burner instead of a sugar-burner. As we've discussed, fat burns at a much steadier rate than carbohydrates, which provide quick bursts of energy followed by the notorious "sugar crash." On a keto diet, you don't experience as many energy surges and lows. In fact, many people report increases in energy levels after following a keto diet for several weeks!

1 Supports Metabolism

2 Blood Sugar Balance

3 Brain Health

4 Mental Focus

5 Uplifted Mood

6 Food Cravings

7 Heart Health

8 Energy Levels

9 Inflammation Response

10 Supports Hormone Balance

What to Expect on the Keto Diet

When you first begin the keto diet, you may experience the side effects that have been nicknamed the "keto flu." This happens because your ketone levels are still rising and you're experiencing withdrawal from carbs and sugar.

Side effects when starting the keto diet can include fatigue, constipation, cravings, headaches, difficulty sleeping, and even bad breath. These are temporary and typically last only one to two weeks. Eating a clean keto diet, drinking lots of water, getting enough electrolytes like salt and magnesium, and consuming exogenous ketones can help reduce the severity of these symptoms. Take a look below at some of the most common keto flu symptoms along with some helpful remedies.

Keto Flu Symptoms and Remedies

1. Low energy

The Problem: If you find that you're feeling fatigued and low on energy no matter how much sleep you're getting after starting to cut carbs, it could be caused by the keto flu.

The Fix: Try giving your energy levels a boost with a small dose of caffeine from ingredients like green tea, matcha, or yerba mate. Alternatively, add a few energizing adaptogens into your daily routine. Maca, ashwagandha, and ginseng are great options to help your body adapt to stress naturally and normalize energy levels.

2. Nausea

The Problem: Nausea is one of the most common—and most unpleasant—side effects of the keto flu.

The Fix: There are plenty of natural remedies that can help soothe the stomach and keep digestive distress at bay. In particular, essential oils like peppermint and ginger can prevent nausea caused by the keto flu. Simply add a few drops to a diffuser or massage a bit onto your stomach or wrists to ward off tummy troubles.

3. Hunger cravings

The Problem: Feeling extra-ravenous between meals? The keto flu may be to blame. Although the keto diet can help cut back on cravings in the long run, it may cause increased hunger when you're first getting started.

The Fix: Try adding a few extra servings of healthy fats and bone broth to your daily diet. These foods can help keep you feeling fuller for longer, without kicking you out of ketosis.

4. Brain-fog

The Problem: This is another symptom that should clear up once you're fully into ketosis. Brain-fog is often characterized by symptoms like forgetfulness, confusion, and lack of focus, and it's a common side effect of the keto flu.

The Fix: Squeezing a bit of light physical activity into your daily routine is an easy way to support mental clarity and battle brain-fog. Adding a few drops of rosemary oil to your diffuser has also been shown to increase memory and enhance concentration.

5. Constipation

The Problem: The keto flu can often throw off regularity, causing side effects like constipation and infrequent bowel movements. Luckily, there are plenty of steps you can take to get your bathroom habits back on track.

The Fix: Drinking more water can help get things moving while also keeping you hydrated. Magnesium also acts as a natural laxative, so try adding more magnesium-rich foods into your diet such as leafy greens and avocado. Probiotics are another simple solution that can give the beneficial bacteria in your gut a boost to promote healthy digestion.

6. Difficulty sleeping

The Problem: Insomnia is a keto flu symptom that can take a serious toll on just about every aspect of health. Not getting enough sleep at night can also worsen other keto flu symptoms, causing a dip in energy levels and contributing to mood swings, brain-fog, and fatigue.

The Fix: Consider adding a collagen supplement to your routine, which contains a mix of amino acids that have been shown to support better sleep, such as glycine. Dabbing a few drops of lavender oil on your wrists before bedtime can also help relieve stress and promote relaxation.

7. Bad breath

The Problem: During the transition to ketosis, many report experiencing "keto

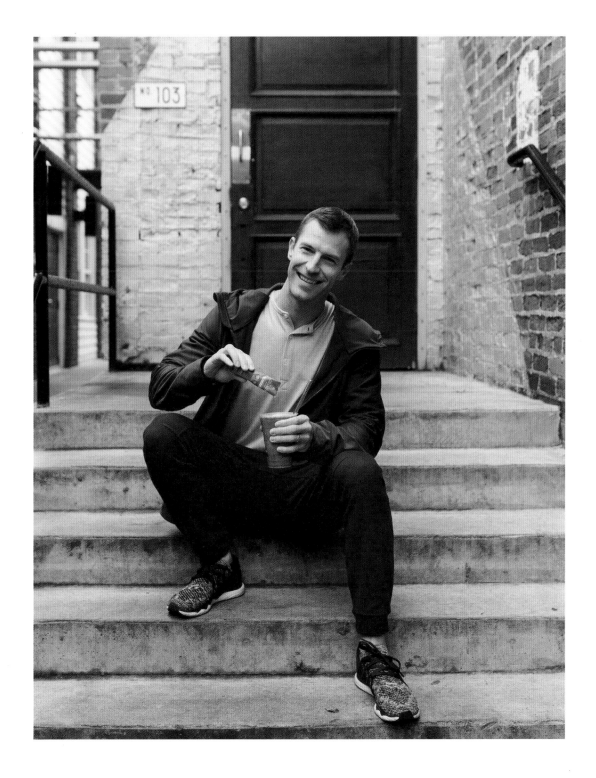

breath," which is caused by the production of acetone, a type of ketone with a fruitlike aroma that tends to leave the body through the breath and urine.

The Fix: Mixing 1 to 2 drops of peppermint oil with a bit of water and swishing it around in your mouth for 30 seconds can help kill bacteria and freshen bad breath. Probiotics have also been shown to support oral hygiene and naturally eliminate odors.

8. Low libido

The Problem: In some cases, cutting back on carbs could cause your sex drive to stall.

The Fix: Try experimenting with some libido-boosting herbs and spices in the kitchen, including nutmeg, saffron, and cloves. Ginseng, maca, and gingko biloba are adaptogens that have also been shown to effectively treat sexual dysfunction in both men and women.

9. Irritability

The Problem: All of us fall into a funk from time to time, but if you're feeling moody, irritable, and depressed just after going keto, it may be a sign of the keto flu.

The Fix: Adding a few mood-elevating herbs into your routine, such as chamomile and holy basil, can help minimize mood swings and prevent irritability. Fish oil can also supply your body with a steady stream of omega-3 fatty acids, which can help bump up brain function and balance your mood.

10. Headaches

The Problem: Headaches can be caused by a number of factors, including stress, depression, or anxiety. Certain dietary or lifestyle changes can also trigger headaches, including starting out on the ketogenic diet.

The Fix: Staying well-hydrated by drinking plenty of water is one of the easiest and most effective ways to treat headaches. You can also try massaging a few drops of lavender oil or peppermint oil onto your temples to increase blood flow and treat headaches naturally.

Headaches

Brain fog

Difficulty sleeping

Bad breath

Hunger cravings

Low energy

Irritability

Nausea

Low libido

Constipation

Following the Keto Diet

Your Macronutrient Ratio on the Keto Diet

The keto diet isn't focused on calorie restriction. Instead, it aims to restrict carbohydrate intake.

Three macronutrients provide us with the calories in our diets: fats, carbohydrates, and proteins. Because fats are your primary energy source on the keto diet, they are the macronutrient that will provide the majority of your daily calories. Healthy fats help support ketone production, decrease your appetite, and keep you from feeling hungry or deprived.

Fats should provide roughly 75% or more of your daily calories. Aim to get about 15 to 20 percent of calories from protein, and just 5 to 10 percent from carbs.

Another number to pay attention to is your net carb intake, meaning the total grams of carbs you eat per day minus the grams of fiber. On a traditional keto diet, the goal is to keep your daily net carb intake below 25 to 30 grams. Some people may be able to stay in ketosis while eating about 50 net grams of carbs per day, so this takes some trial and error. Achieving this means that grains, most fruits, starches, and sugary snacks are off-limits. (See 3 Steps to Adjusting Your Macros for more information.)

The more you restrict your carb intake, the quicker you'll enter ketosis. Some find that limiting carb consumption to just 15 grams per day for the first two weeks kickstarts ketosis and minimizes keto flu symptoms (see more on page 17).

For most people, it is appropriate to stay in ketosis for a duration of two to six months (or potentially longer, if you're working with a doctor). In order to maintain results, you may choose to try approaches like keto cycling or carb-cycling long term, which involves eating very low-carb most days of the week, but intentionally increasing carbs on other days to restore glycogen reserves.

Calculating your macronutrient intake is a key component of the ketogenic diet. It's essential for helping your body reach ketosis while also providing it with the nutrients that it needs.

Here are three simple steps to adjust your macronutrient intake when going keto.

1. Decrease Carb Consumption

Cutting down on carbs is the first step for going keto. Restricting carb consumption switches your body into a state of ketosis, flipping it from a sugar-burner to a fat-burner by depriving it of glucose, which is its main source of fuel.

Most people can reach ketosis by limiting carb intake to 30–50 grams of net carbs per day. Net carbs are calculated by subtracting the grams of fiber from the total grams of carbs in a food. For instance, if a food contains 10 grams of carbs and 3 grams of fiber, it would have just 7 grams of net carbs.

To keep carb intake in check, stick to high-fiber, low-carb ingredients like non-starchy vegetables and low-sugar fruits. Steer clear of foods like grains, dairy, and sugary snacks, which can quickly catapult you beyond your carb count for the day.

2. Monitor Protein Intake

Getting the right ratio of protein in your diet is also crucial for maintaining ketosis. If you eat too much protein, your body can start converting it into glucose, stalling ketosis, and setting back your progress. Conversely, not getting enough protein can stall muscle growth and weaken immune function.

As a general rule of thumb, approximately 15–20 percent of your total daily calories should come from protein. This means that if you're eating 2,000 calories per day, 300–400 calories should come from high-quality protein foods. To convert protein calories into grams, simply divide by 4. For example, 300–400 calories of protein per day translates to 75–100 grams of protein.

Be sure to select high-quality protein foods from sources like grass-fed meat, free-range poultry, and wild-caught seafood. Other foods like eggs, fermented soy products, nuts, and seeds can also provide an added dose of protein to your diet.

3. Increase Healthy Fat Consumption

Bumping up your intake of heart-healthy fats is a crucial component of the ketogenic diet. Not eating enough fat can impair your body's ability to produce ketones, leaving energy levels low.

About 70–80 percent of your total daily calories should come from fat. For example, on a diet of 2,000 calories per day, 1,400–1,600 calories should come from heart-healthy fats. Divide this number by 9 to estimate how many grams of fat you should consume daily. In this example, 1,400–1,600 calories divided by 9 yields 155–178 grams of fat.

Loading up on the wrong types of fat can be harmful to health, which is why it's essential to stick to heart-healthy sources instead. Olive oil, avocados, coconut oil, MCT oil, nuts, seeds, and grass-fed butter are all examples of nutritious fats that can fit seamlessly into a ketogenic diet.

Following the Keto Diet

The Keto Diet Foods List

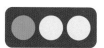

Foods to eat anytime

- **Healthy fats:** olive oil, coconut oil, grass-fed butter, ghee, palm oil, avocado oil, avocado, MCT oil, lard, chicken fat, duck fat

- **Quality protein:** grass-fed meat, pasture-raised poultry, cage-free eggs, all types of wild-caught fish and seafood (such as tuna, trout, anchovies, bass, flounder, mackerel, salmon, sardines), organ meats like liver, turkey or beef jerky

- **Non-starchy vegetables:** broccoli, cauliflower, Brussels sprouts, and other cruciferous veggies, all types of leafy greens (such as spinach, dandelion and beet greens, collards, mustard, turnip, arugula, chicory, endive, escarole, fennel, radicchio, and kale), asparagus, cucumber, celery, mushrooms, bell peppers, zucchini, tomatoes (be careful to limit sweeter veggies like potatoes, butternut squash, beets)

- **Nuts and seeds:** almonds, walnuts, cashews, sunflower seeds, pistachios, chestnuts, pumpkin seeds, nut and seed butters, chia seeds (limit your intake to about ¼ cup per day, or 2 tablespoons of nut/seed butter)

- **Low-carb beverages:** water, seltzer, herbal tea, black/green tea, black coffee, bone broth

- **Herbs and spices:** all types of fresh or dried herbs/spices such as cinnamon, basil, rosemary, thyme, turmeric, ginger, cilantro, red pepper

- **Condiments:** hot sauce, apple cider vinegar and other vinegars, unsweetened mustard, soy sauce, lemon/lime juice, cocoa powder, stevia extract, vanilla extract

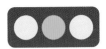

Foods to eat occasionally

- **Full-fat dairy products:** heavy cream, sour cream, organic cheeses, and, in small amounts, full-fat/unsweetened yogurt, kefir, milk
- **Medium-starchy vegetables:** sweet peas, artichokes, okra, carrots, beets
- **Beans and legumes:** chickpeas, kidney beans, lima beans, black beans, pinto beans, lentils, hummus
- **Fruit:** berries, including blueberries, strawberries, blackberries, raspberries
- **Condiments:** No-sugar-added ketchup or salsa, low-sugar salad dressings, pickles, monk fruit
- **Drinks:** fresh vegetable juices, unsweetened coconut or almond milk, water flavored with lemon or lime juice

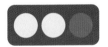

Foods to avoid

- Anything made with added sugar, including white, brown, cane, raw, and confectioners' sugar, plus syrups like maple, honey, and agave
- All drinks high in sugar
- Foods made with any grains or grain flour, including all whole grains and white/wheat flour
- Corn and all products containing corn
- Potatoes and other starchy veggies (may be appropriate in very small quantities)
- Conventional dairy products, including most yogurts, ice cream, milk
- **Snacks:** granola bars, nearly all protein bars or meal replacements (low-carb bars tend to have unhealthy artificial ingredients), most canned soups, many condiments, and many prepackaged meals
- Most fruit (berries can be eaten in small quantities)

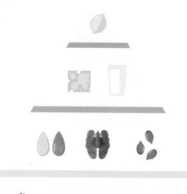

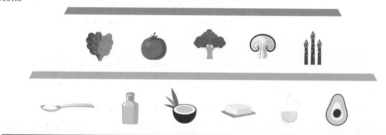

Low-Carb Fruits

Blackberries
Blueberries
Grapefruit
Lemons
Limes
Raspberries
Strawberries

Full-Fat Dairy

Unsweetened yogurt
Kefir
Raw milk
Healthy cheeses
  feta, goat, cottage,
  ricotta

Nut and Seeds

Almonds
Walnuts
Cashews
Pistachios
Chestnuts
Pumpkin seeds
Chia seeds
Flax seeds
Sunflower seeds
Nut butters
Seed butters

Healthy Fats

Grass-fed butter
Ghee
Coconut oil
MCT oil
Extra virgin olive oil
Flax oil
Avocados

Non-Starchy Vegetables

Asparagus
Broccoli
Brussels sprouts
Cabbage
Celery
Cucumber
Leafy greens
Mushrooms

Seaweed
  nori, wakame,
  kombu, dulse
Spinach
Spirulina
Tomato
Zucchini
Herbs and spices

Protein Foods

Cage-free eggs
Grass-fed meat
  beef, lamb, goat, veal, venison
Organic poultry
  chicken, turkey, goose, duck
Wild-caught fish
  salmon, mackerel, sardines,
  anchovies, tuna
Free-range organ meats,
such as liver

Easy Keto Food Swaps

Now that you know which foods are keto-friendly and which aren't, here are eight simple swaps to help you get started.

1. Swap pasta for zucchini noodles

Regular pasta is high in carbs and calories, and it is lacking in many of the nutrients that your body needs. Next time the spaghetti cravings strike, try making zucchini noodles instead. Cup for cup, zucchini noodles contain about one-tenth of the calories and carbs of regular pasta. What's more, zucchinis are loaded with important nutrients, including vitamin A, manganese, vitamin C, and potassium.

2. Swap granola bars for bone broth protein bars

Most granola bars are packed full of preservatives, fillers, and artificial flavors. Many even contain more sugar per serving than some candy bars. For this reason, bone broth protein bars make a much better choice. In addition to providing plenty of protein, healthy fats, and fiber, they also supply a hearty dose of collagen, which can help support joint, immune, skin, and gut health.

3. Swap protein powder for collagen protein

Many types of protein powder are made from whey, which is a type of natural sugar found in milk. Although whey protein is a popular post-workout snack, it's also high in carbs and may not be the best choice on a ketogenic diet. Collagen protein, on the other hand, is high in protein and carb-free, meaning it can help boost muscle growth without kicking you out of ketosis.

4. Swap sugar for stevia

Cutting down on sugar consumption is a key component of the ketogenic diet. Fortunately, switching to stevia can help satisfy your sweet tooth without all the side effects of sugar. Stevia is a natural, non-nutritive sweetener that provides the same sweetness as regular sugar, but with none of the carbs and calories. Try using a pinch of stevia to sweeten up your favorite keto-friendly hot beverages, smoothies, or baked goods.

5. Swap buns for lettuce wrap

Using a lettuce wrap instead of a bun is an easy way to give your next burger a tasty, low-carb twist. Besides being virtually free of carbohydrates, swapping in a lettuce wrap can also slash the amount of sodium and calories in your meal. Plus, eating lettuce is a great way to squeeze an extra dose of vitamin A, vitamin C, and fiber into your diet.

6. Swap conventional milk for coconut milk

If you're looking to bump up your intake of heart-healthy fats, try trading your conventional milk for coconut milk. Coconut milk is brimming with medium-chain triglycerides (MCTs), which are easily broken down in the liver to give your body a quick burst of energy. MCTs are also converted into ketones, which can help speed up your transition into ketosis.

7. Swap baking flour for almond flour

Almond flour is a pantry staple in any low-carb kitchen. It contains many fewer carbs than regular flour, but significantly more protein, healthy fats, and fiber. It's also gluten-free and rich in vitamins and minerals, making it a great addition to keto flatbreads, pies, waffles, pancakes, and other low-carb treats.

8. Swap bean dip for guacamole

Bean dip is a popular dipping sauce, typically made with a mix of refried beans and other ingredients such as sour cream, cheese, and canned chiles. Sadly, it's not particularly healthy. Guacamole and tahini are two great, keto-friendly alternatives to bean dip. Made from avocados and sesame seeds respectively, both are high in healthy fats and an assortment of important vitamins and minerals. Each can also be made at home using real, whole food ingredients rather than products that have been heavily processed and refined.

A number of different iterations of the ketogenic diet exist, but all have this in common: you eat plenty of fats while also drastically reducing the amount of carbs you eat. They differ in terms of the quality of foods that are emphasized, the amount of animal products (like meat and fish) that are included, and the sustainability of the diet. Here are some different takes on the classic keto diet.

- **Clean keto diet:** Focuses on minimally processed whole foods, including plenty of healthy fats/oils, quality meats/protein in moderation, and lots of non-starchy vegetables, herbs, spices, bone broth, and probiotic foods.

- **Modified keto diet:** Similar to a modified Atkins diet, this variation includes a bit more protein and carbs than a traditional keto diet. It's still high in fat and low in carbs, but it allows for more flexibility and food variety. It may not be easy to stay in ketosis while following this modified plan, but some feel it's a healthy and sustainable way to eat long term.

- **Ketotarian diet:** This is a keto diet with a mostly plant-based or pescatarian twist. It's a great fit for people who want to experience the benefits of keto on a mostly plant-based diet, meaning minimal meat, dairy, eggs, fish, etc.

- **Eco-keto diet:** "Eco-Keto" is a catchy way of describing an eco-friendly, ketogenic diet. Most people think of eco-keto as a totally plant-based, aka vegan, keto diet. Raising and transporting livestock, especially beef, requires more food, water, land, and energy than plant foods do, which is why filling up on more plant proteins (like tofu and protein powders) can be a more ecologically sustainable way to follow the keto diet.

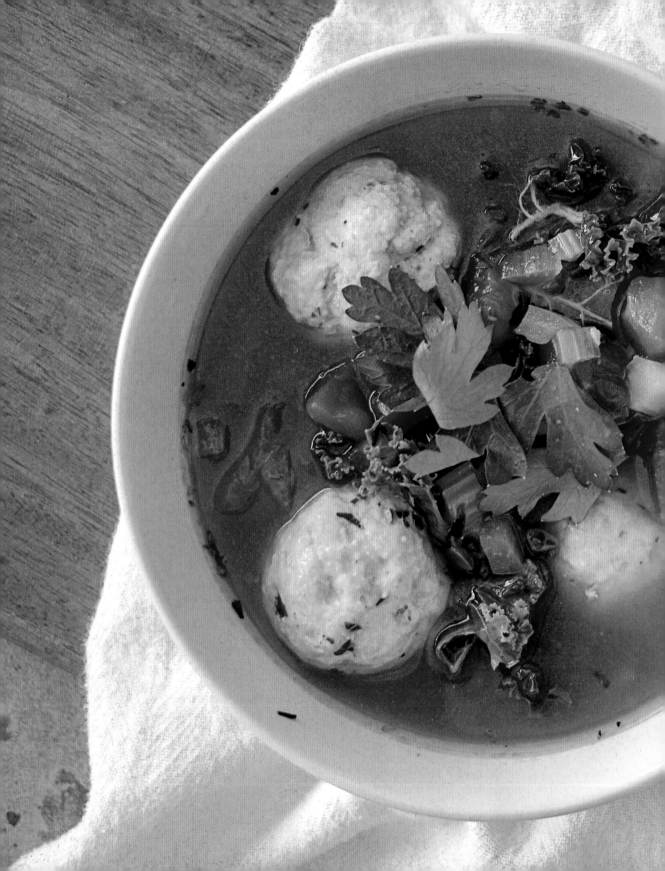

Part II

Practical Keto Living

The Keto Guide to Cooking Fats

Staying in ketosis requires you to get 70 percent or more of your daily calories from fat. This means that cooking oils and other healthy fats should be primary ingredients in all of your meals and snacks.

So, which fats and oils qualify as healthy? The best cooking oils and fats to incorporate into your diet include:

- Olive oil (especially extra virgin olive oil)
- Coconut oil
- MCT oil
- Avocado oil
- Grass-fed butter
- Grass-fed ghee
- Grapeseed oil
- Walnut oil
- Sesame oil
- Tallow
- Other quality nut and seed oils such as hazelnut, pistachio, flaxseed, hemp

To add more healthy fat to your diet, look for ingredients that are unprocessed and naturally high in fats. Aside from cooking oils, other healthy fat-filled foods to fill up on include avocados, nuts, and seeds, plus animal products like fish, meat, eggs, and dairy.

Choosing Cooking Fats

Here are some tips for choosing the best cooking fats:

- **Aim for a mix of different fats.** This includes unsaturated fats like olive oil, avocado oil, and other high-quality nut and seed oils. But don't be afraid of saturated fats, which are found in butter, coconut oil, and also animal products like dairy products (cream, buttermilk, etc.).

- **Avoid highly-processed vegetable oils.** "Vegetable oils" refer to oils that come from plant sources. They are commonly made with chemical solvents and found in many packaged snacks like chips, crackers, and baked goods. While some consider canola oil a healthy choice, canola oil in the United

States and many other nations tends to be highly processed and "cold-pressed" or unprocessed canola oil is difficult to find.

- **Stay away from artery-clogging trans fats, butter substitute spreads, and margarine.** These items should be avoided at all costs. They are commonly used to fry cheap, processed foods and can be found in many fast foods and processed baked goods.

- **Use toasted nut and seed oils.** Selections such as walnut, pistachio, flaxseed, hemp, and sesame oils add healthy fats and big flavor to your meals. But they have low smoke points, so don't cook with them at high temps (or at all).

All About Smoke Points

An oil's smoke point is the temperature at which the oil starts burning and smoking. In order to preserve the healthy fats found in quality oils, you need to keep the oil's smoke point in mind. Exceeding it will damage the oil's fatty acids, burn off important minerals, and ruin the flavor of your meal. So when you're cooking at high temps—to sear meat, for instance—be sure to use an oil with a high smoke point. Keep these tips in mind:

- The best choice of cooking oil depends on the cooking method you're using.

- When frying, sautéing, or roasting, select a cooking fat with a high smoke point, such as avocado oil or ghee.

- Cooking oils with a low smoke point can oxidize and break down under high heat, leading to the formation of harmful, disease-causing free radicals.

- Cooking oils with a low smoke point, like extra virgin olive oil or walnut oil, should be used raw to add calories and flavor to salads, veggies, dips, spreads, and dressings.

SMOKE POINTS AT A GLANCE

Here are the smoke points of cooking fats and oils from lowest to highest:

- Butter (300 to 350°F)

- Walnut oil (320°F)

- MCT oil (320°F)

- Olive oil (320 to 420°F, depending on the variety)

- Coconut oil (350°F)

- Grapeseed oil (420°F)

- Tallow (420°F)

- Palm oil (450°F)

- Ghee (485°F)

- Avocado oil (520°F)

Helpful Tips:

Low- or no-heat cooking fats/oils: butter, MCT oil, extra virgin olive oil, sesame oil, walnut oil, hemp oil, flaxseed oil, and most other other nut/seed oils

High-heat-friendly cooking fats/oils (for grilling, roasting, frying): grapeseed oil, avocado oil, grass-fed ghee, tallow, palm oil

Using the Best Cooking Oils and Fats

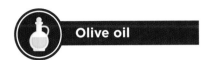

Olive oil contains a large amount of monounsaturated fats and some polyunsaturated fatty acids. Consumption has been linked to lower blood pressure, reduced cholesterol levels, cognitive health, and improved blood vessel function, among other benefits. Extra virgin varieties of olive oil have the highest nutrient content and no chemicals are involved in the manufacturing process. When shopping, look for a seal from the International Olive Oil Council and check the harvesting date on the label.

- **Smoke point:** 325 to 405°F

- **When to use it:** Use as a "finishing oil" for flavor and for low- and medium-heat cooking. It's perfect in vinaigrettes, salad dressings, or marinades; for drizzling over veggies; or for enhancing the flavor of other cooked foods.

- **When to avoid using it:** Due to its low smoke point, olive oil isn't recommended for cooking at high temperatures. Avoid it when roasting, baking, or frying.

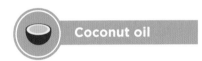

The high saturated fat content of coconut oil makes it useful for increasing your good cholesterol levels and promoting heart health. It also provides easily absorbed medium-chain fats, has anti-inflammatory properties, and is beneficial for gut health. Choose extra virgin coconut oil if possible.

- **Smoke point:** 350°F

- **When to use it:** Coconut oil is great for roasting at low temperatures, baking, and as an ingredient in smoothies/shakes or coffee. It can easily be substituted for other oils or butters using a 1:1 ratio in most recipes.

- **When to avoid using it:** Coconut oil is solid at room temperature, so it's not the best choice when you need a healthy fat in liquid form for drizzling on salad. Like olive oil, it has a relatively low smoke point, so avoid using it when roasting or frying at high temperatures. And remember that it may add a mild coconut flavor to recipes.

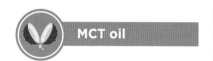 **MCT oil**

MCTs (medium-chain triglycerides) are a form of saturated fat that is easily digested, may help increase energy, and helps you feel full. MCT oil is not typically used for cooking because it's more expensive than other oils, although it can be used in place of coconut oil if desired. It's usually treated more like a supplement than a cooking fat.

- **Smoke point:** 320°F

- **When to use it:** MCT oil can be used in salad dressings, added to smoothies and shakes, or used to replace about one-third of the coconut oil in recipes (1 part MCT oil to 2 parts coconut oil), such as when baking.

- **When to avoid using it:** MCT oil may add a "greasy" quality to recipes, so it generally isn't used for cooking. Avoid using it at very high temperatures, such as when roasting or frying.

 Avocado oil

Avocado oil has a mild taste that won't over-power dishes the way some other oils may, plus it has a high smoke point, which means it holds its nutritional value better than some other oils. Avocado oil also provides antioxidants, vitamin E, and healthy monounsaturated fats. It also has a pleasant creamy quality.

- **Smoke point:** 520°F

- **When to use it:** Avocado oil is perfect for grilling, roasting, or pan-frying. Because it remains liquid at room temperature, it's also a good choice to drizzle on salads, sandwiches, or veggies. It can also be used to add creaminess to dips like guacamole and can replace mayonnaise in certain recipes.

- **When to avoid using it:** Avocado oil is very versatile, and there aren't many cases when it ought to be avoided. It tends to be expensive, however, so it's not always the best option if you're on a budget.

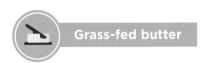
Grass-fed butter

Butter provides omega-6 and omega-3 fats, and even some fat-soluble vitamins like vitamins E and A, plus trace minerals. Opt for real butter—preferably raw butter or butter sourced from grass-fed, organic cows—over lower-calorie substitutes.

- **Smoke point:** 300 to 350°F

- **When to use it:** Use butter for making baked goods, cooking eggs, or as a spread on keto bread or pancakes. It's also delicious tossed in roasted veggies.

- **When to avoid using it:** Avoid using butter for high-heat cooking such as frying or roasting.

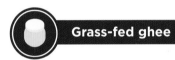
Grass-fed ghee

Ghee is a type of clarified butter that's simmered to bring out a naturally nutty flavor. It has a higher smoke point than regular butter, making it ideal for cooking at high temperatures, plus it's more easily tolerated by people with dairy/lactose intolerance because it's lactose- and casein-free. When shopping, look for organic or grass-fed cultured ghee.

- **Smoke point:** 485°F

- **When to use it:** Use ghee for sautéing veggies and meats, and baking. You can use ghee in place of butter in any cooking or baking recipe.

- **When to avoid using it:** Ghee is versatile and easy to use in most situations, but it can be harder to find and more expensive than butter.

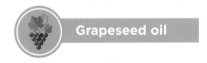
Grapeseed oil

Grapeseed oil is high in polyunsaturated fats, which means it should not be used for high-heat cooking. It's also a great source of vitamin E.

- **Smoke point:** 420°F

- **When to use it:** Grapeseed oil is great for making salad dressings, dips, or baked goods.

- **When to avoid using it:** Grapeseed oil should be avoided when frying, roasting at high temps, or grilling.

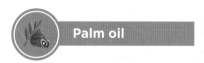 **Palm oil**

High in saturated fat and semi-solid at room temperature, palm oil can be used as a substitute for trans fats in baking. It works well as a frying oil because it has a relatively high smoke point and neutral flavor.

- **Smoke point:** 450°F

- **When to use it:** Palm oil is ideal for frying and baking.

- **When to avoid using it:** Avoid using palm oil in dressings or if you're looking for unique flavor.

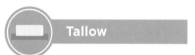 **Tallow**

Tallow is made from animal fat (usually beef fat) and remains solid at room temperature. Some see it as a hybrid of coconut oil and butter. It contains mostly saturated fat but also some monounsaturated fat. It can be used at relatively high temps and has a mild flavor, making it a good alternative to coconut oil or ghee.

- **Smoke point:** 420°F

- **When to use it:** Use tallow for pan frying, deep frying, or roasting meat or veggies.

- **When to avoid using it:** Tallow isn't a good option for making dressings, baking, or when you're looking for light and unique flavor.

 Walnut oil

Walnut oil is a good source of omega-3 and omega-6 fats, plus it provides an appealing flavor. Because it has a low smoke point, it's best for drizzling on foods rather than cooking.

- **Smoke point:** 320°F

- **When to use it:** Add some to keto pancakes or muffins, stir it into coffee or a keto smoothie, or incorporate it in dressings/vinaigrettes.

- **When to avoid using it:** Walnut oil's low smoke point makes it a bad choice for high-heat cooking.

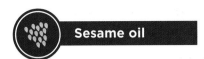 **Sesame oil**

Sesame oil contains both monounsaturated and polyunsaturated fatty acids and has a high smoke point. It also adds lots of unique flavor (especially if it's toasted sesame oil), even in small amounts.

- **Smoke point:** 410°F

- **When to use it:** Use sesame oil in marinades, sautés, roasts, stir-fries, and for finishing meals with big flavor.

- **When to avoid using it:** Avoid sesame oil when frying, baking, or whenever you don't want to add sesame flavor.

Dining Out on Keto

Thanks to the growing popularity of the keto diet, there are now plenty of healthy keto options available at most restaurants, even at places you wouldn't expect, like some fast-food joints.

While preparing most of your meals at home is the best way to stick to your plan, to ensure you're consuming high-quality ingredients, and to see progress, you still need to live your life and dine out here and there. By choosing what you order wisely and making some simple substitutions, you should be able to enjoy meals out without sabotaging your diet.

Key Principles for Dining Out

Follow these nine principles when eating out to make sure you stay in ketosis.

1. Check out menus ahead of time; this way you can choose a restaurant that you know offers something keto-friendly.

2. Don't be afraid to ask to customize your order. Request extra grilled chicken on your salad with veggies for example, or salad dressing on the side.

3. Focus on healthy fats (like olive oil, ghee, and butter), vegetables, and simply cooked protein.

4. Try to dine at places that offer meat that has been raised sustainably and humanely. Whenever possible, choose meat/poultry that is 100 percent organic grass-fed, free-range, or pasture-raised. Fish should ideally be wild-caught.

5. Avoid anything fried or breaded. Go for the grilled, roasted, blackened, or baked proteins.

6. Skip the bread basket, buns, biscuits, and rolls. Ask for extra lettuce, tomato, onions, and pickles instead. You can make your own lettuce wrap with any protein.

7. Want to add more flavor to your meals? Try using approved condiments and seasonings, such as salt and pepper, vinegars, hot sauce, unsweetened

mustard, pico de gallo, lime or lemon juice, basil, garlic powder, hot peppers, oregano, and thyme.

8. Don't drink your calories. Stick with plain water, seltzer, unsweetened coffee, or teas.

9. Just say no to the dessert menu. This way you aren't tempted.

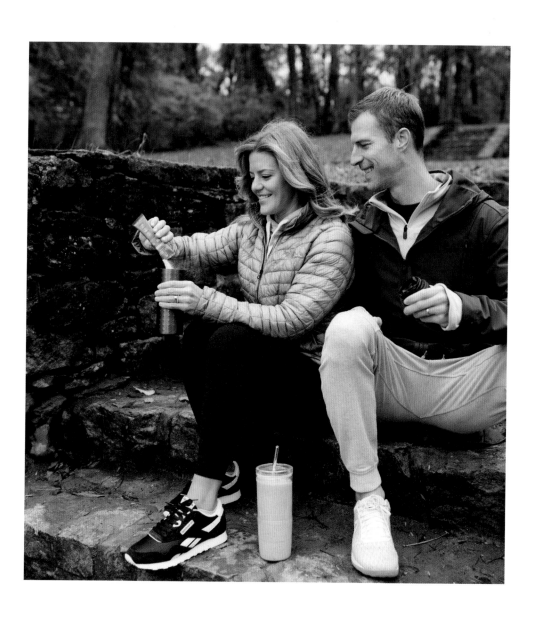

Top Keto-Friendly Options

Here are some tips on what to look for when dining out at different types of restaurants.

- At any salad joint, order a salad with leafy greens, cruciferous veggies, celery, cucumber, fresh herbs, avocado, egg, and/or protein. For dressing, choose olive oil, lemon juice, or fresh squeezed lime juice.

- At cafes or sports bars, when in doubt, choose a salad or side of cooked non-starchy veggies with a protein. Skip the standard salad dressing and request plain olive oil and vinegar, or avocado oil instead.

- At a Mexican restaurant, choose a salad with grass-fed beef and fajita-style veggies. You can also add avocado and a small amount of black or lima beans, salsa, or sour cream.

- At an Italian or Greek restaurant, look for fish options that aren't fried or breaded, and request extra veggies.

- At a Japanese, Chinese, or Thai restaurant, skip the rice and ask for stir-fries with extra veggies and light sauce, or sashimi-style fish instead of sushi.

High-Carb Options to Avoid

Regardless of where you're dining, make sure to avoid these foods at all costs, They'll knock you right out of ketosis!

- Sandwiches and burgers served on bread/buns
- Pasta dishes
- Pizza
- Tacos or burritos served in tortillas/flour wraps
- Egg sandwiches or omelettes served on bread/biscuits/rolls
- Processed meats like bacon and sausage (these may be low in carbs but are still unhealthy)
- Fried chicken, chicken cutlets, chicken fingers, and most chicken wings
- Mozzarella sticks, quesadillas, and potato skins

- Salads topped with sugary dressing and dried fruit
- Dishes made with sweet marinades or sauces, glazes, reductions, BBQ sauce, and lots of ketchup
- Sweetened beverages, like alcohol, soda, juice, ice tea, or coffee drinks like lattes
- All desserts, including ice cream, cake, and cookies

Smart Swaps and Substitutions

Now that you know what to avoid, here are some easy swaps you can make while dining out.

Instead of this: hamburger on a bun
Order this: hamburger with no bun (no ketchup), served over greens or in a lettuce wrap

Instead of this: pasta dish with chicken
Order this: chicken with an extra side of vegetables or salad

Instead of this: salad with cranberries, candied nuts, cheese, and sweet dressing
Order this: salad with a protein and fresh vegetables, dressed with olive oil and vinegar, plus a bit of nuts and cheese. Go light on the cheese and skip the croutons, fruit, and any sweet add-ons.

Instead of this: sides like French fries, baked potato, rice, bread, or pasta
Order this: extra vegetables dressed with butter or oil, or a side salad

Instead of this: chicken cutlet sandwich or chicken fingers
Order this: grilled chicken with extra greens, avocado if available, a bit of cheese, tomato, and pickles

Instead of this: fish tacos in flour or corn tortillas
Order this: grilled or blackened fish with extra slaw, salad, and fresh lemon/lime juice. Ask for your meal fajita style, so you can skip the tortilla but keep all the sides.

Instead of this: chicken or steak burrito with rice and beans
Order this: burrito bowl served over lettuce, with protein, pico de gallo, and guacamole. Ask for a smaller portion of black beans and cheese.

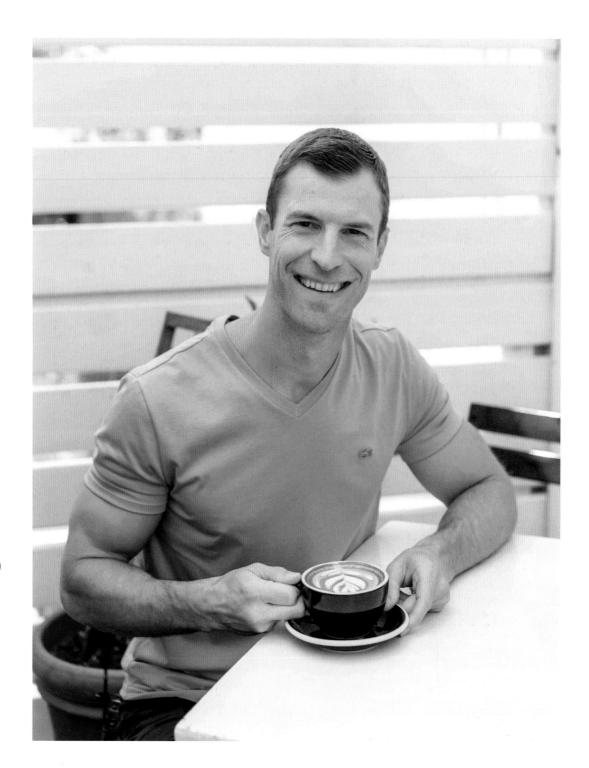

Instead of this: pizza
Order this: meat and cheese board, served with nuts, olives, and pickled vegetables topped with olive oil

Instead of this: orange chicken, sweet and sour beef, or other sweetened/breaded dishes at Chinese restaurants
Order this: chicken or beef stir-fry with veggies and no rice (ask for light sauce)

Instead of this: bacon, egg, and cheese on a roll/biscuit
Order this: veggie omelet (no potatoes/hash browns), or two fried eggs with cheese, tomato, and avocado (skip the biscuit or bread)

Instead of this: sweetened coffee drinks like a frappuccino, latte, or cappuccino
Order this: black coffee with a tablespoon of coconut oil, grass-fed butter, or even collagen protein powder mixed in (if you have this on hand).

DINING OUT IN A HURRY!

Fast food isn't something you want to make a habit of relying on; however, sometimes we find ourselves in a pinch with limited options. When visiting a fast-food restaurant or chain, chances are you can find a low-carb salad on the menu along with healthy additions available like grilled chicken, fresh veggies, or avocado.

Look for options such as oven-roasted chicken, steak and cheese, roast beef or turkey breast, tuna salad, egg salad, or chicken salad (these can often be bought by the pound). To make salads more filling, load up on non-starchy veggies, like peppers, tomatoes, radishes, and cucumber.

Depending on where you live, some of the best places to order keto "fast food" include:

- Panera Bread
- Chipotle
- Chopt
- Elevation Burger
- Wendy's
- Subway
- McDonald's
- Carl's Jr.
- Chick-fil-A
- Starbucks
- Jersey Mikes
- Taco Bell
- Five Guys Burgers
- Burger King
- Smashburger

Top 10 Keto Supplements Guide

In order to get the most out of the keto diet, you not only need to eat the right foods, but also incorporate keto-supportive supplements. Here are my most recommended keto supplements that will help support your efforts while you're on a keto diet.

Exogenous Ketones

What it is:

- Ketone supplements

- Usually contain the ketone beta hydroxybutyrate (BHB), which is great for both transitioning to a keto diet and maintaining the state of ketosis

How it works:

- Used to mimic or amplify the positive effects of calorie restriction or keto diets

- Should also contain MCTs and organic adaptogenic herbs with antioxidant properties (which support metabolism, boost energy, and promote mental focus)

Collagen Protein

What it is:

- A must-have supplement for those following the keto diet

- Provides a unique blend of amino acids and other compounds associated with healthy joint function

- Should feature high-quality protein and fat

How it works:

- Boosts mind and muscle power

- Helps to support healthy joints, promote healthy skin, and support a healthy gut

SBO Probiotics

What it is:

- Soil-based organisms (SBO) are probiotic strains that naturally occur in soil and are often found in organic fruit and vegetables

- Should feature microorganisms that help populate the guts of people with diets rich in fats and proteins and lower in carbohydrates

- Should contain at least 20 billion CFUs (colony forming units) per serving

How it works:

- Supports a healthy GI system, healthy gut flora, healthy immune system, and healthy intestinal function

- Helps to promote regular bowel function and maintain an already healthy immune system

Lipase Digestive Enzymes

What it is:

- Lipases break down fat into its component parts

- Should contain specifically designed lipase digestive enzymes, heavier on fat-digesting and protein-digesting enzymes

How it works:

- Helps to support proper digestion

- Should include a shelf-stable probiotic to support overall digestive health

Multivitamin

What it is:

- A whole-foods multivitamin that features both fat-soluble and water-soluble vitamins

- Should contain an array of enzyme-activated minerals and probiotic-fermented nutrients

How it works:

- Helps to ensure your body gets the vitamins and minerals it needs, which is crucial for keto dieters

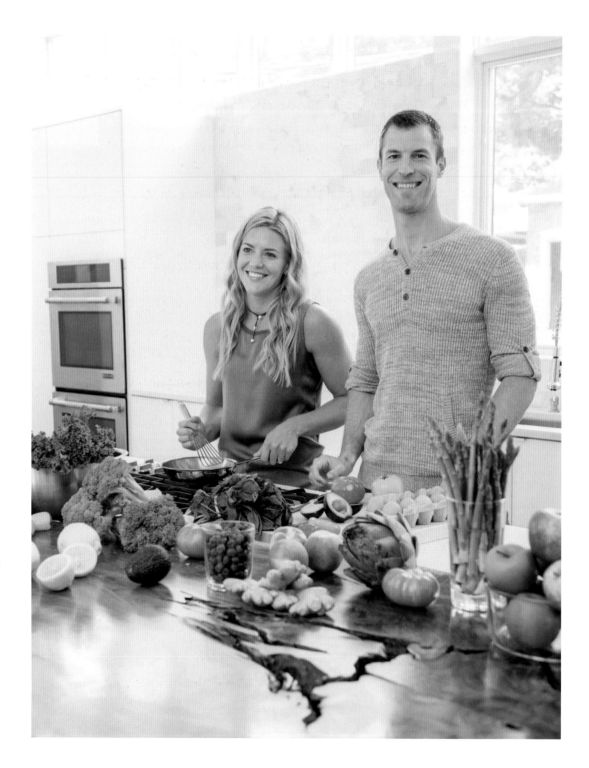

Organic Greens Powder

What it is:

- Powdered supplement made from powerful superfoods and organic whole fruits, vegetables, and herbs

How it works:

- Should also contain probiotics and enzymes to support healthy nutrient absorption and digestion

- Provides the extra boost of energy you need while following a keto diet

Ashwagandha

What it is:

- One of the therapeutic herbs most utilized in Ayurvedic treatments

How it works:

- Supports mental focus and clarity, a healthy mood, and energy levels

- Contains adaptogenic properties, which help to fight stress by lowering cortisol levels

- Can help to promote weight loss, increase energy, and boost metabolism

- Should be a full-spectrum fermented blend to support your keto lifestyle

Turmeric

What it is:

- The dried root of the *Curcuma longa* plant and the main spice used in curry

How it works:

- Contains the active ingredient curcumin, which helps to support healthy inflammation response

MCT Oil

What it is:

- Oil made from medium-chain fats extracted from certain vegetable oils (coconut and palm kernel)

How it works:

- Easily broken down in the liver, provides your body with a quick and convenient burst of energy

- Can also be converted into ketones, helping you reach ketosis faster and bypass keto flu symptoms

- Should be organic and sourced from coconuts to add an energizing dose of healthy fats to your diet

Cannabidiol (CBD) Oil

What it is:

- A non-psychoactive compound in the marijuana plant linked to benefits ranging from pain relief to reduced anxiety

- Should have a certificate of analysis, or COA, which means it's been tested for contaminants and meets specific standards for quality and purity

How it works:

- May also help amplify the effects of the ketogenic diet to reduce inflammation and boost brain health

1. Exogenous Ketones
2. Collagen Protein
3. SBO Probiotics
4. Lipase Digestive Enzymes
5. Multivitamin
6. Organic Greens Powder
7. Ashwagandha
8. Turmeric
9. MCT Oil
10. CBD Oil

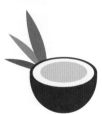

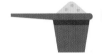

Top 10 Keto Supplements Guide

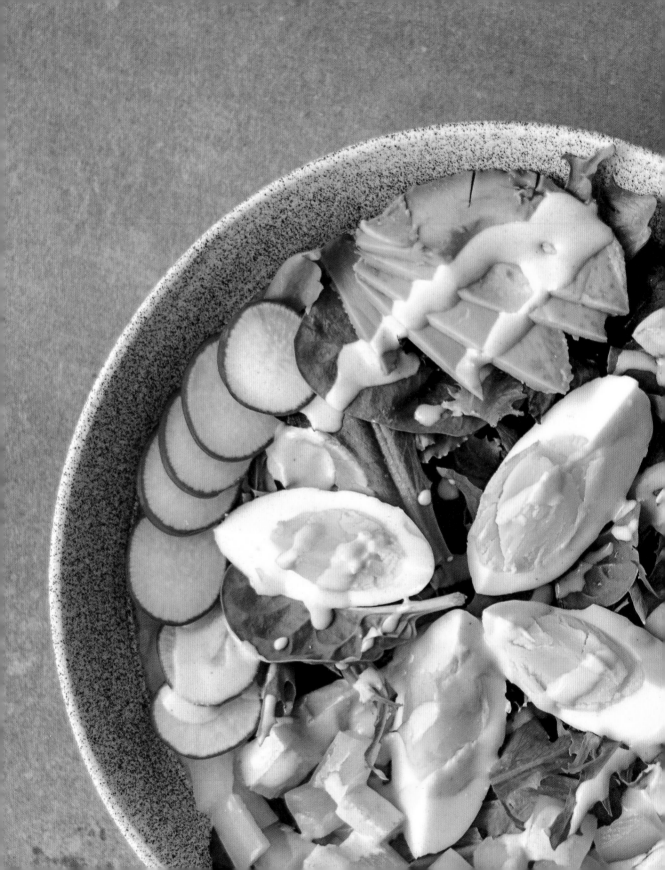

Part III

Keto Diet Recipes

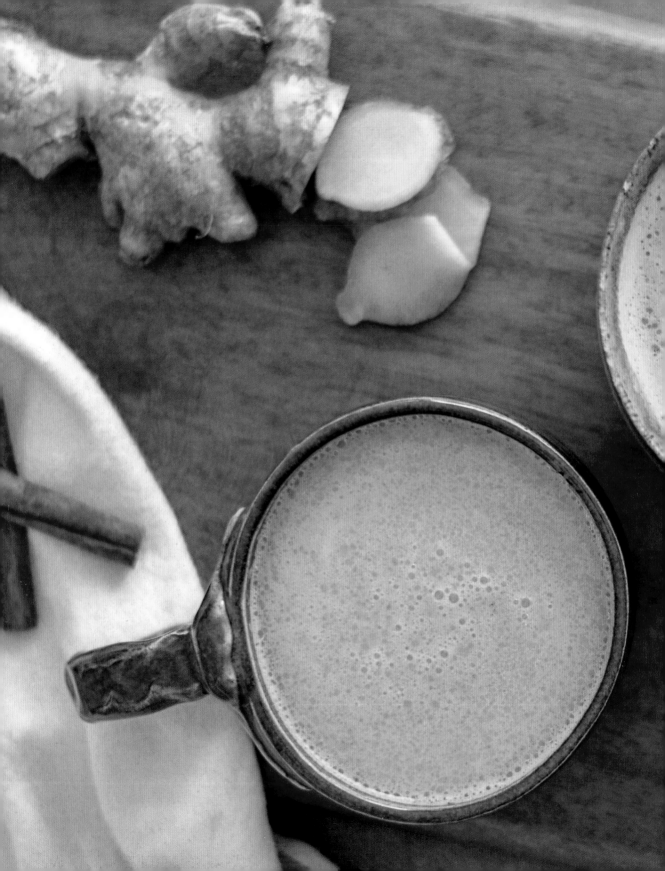

Smoothies
and
Drinks

AB&J Milkshake

Serves: 2 / Time: 5 minutes

INGREDIENTS

½ avocado

3 tablespoons almond butter

1 cup unsweetened almond milk

4 to 6 ice cubes

½ cup strawberries

Juice of ½ lime

1 scoop keto collagen powder (vanilla)

DIRECTIONS

Place all the ingredients in a high-speed blender and blend until smooth.

Nutrition information per serving: *360 calories, 30.6 g fat, 5.8 g saturated fat, 14.1 g protein, 11.4 g carbohydrate, 6.3 g fiber, 165 mg sodium*

Anti-inflammatory Ginger–Apple Cider Vinegar Drink

Serves: 6 / Time: 5 minutes

INGREDIENTS

3 cups filtered water

¼ cup organic apple cider vinegar

1½ inches fresh ginger, peeled

½ inch fresh turmeric, peeled

Juice of 1 lemon

Pinch of freshly ground black pepper

DIRECTIONS

Place all the ingredients in a high-speed blender. Blend on high for 20 to 30 seconds, or until the ginger and turmeric are blended and well incorporated.

Store in an airtight glass jar in the refrigerator for up to a week. If separation occurs, gently shake or stir it.

Nutrition information per serving: *5 calories, 0 g fat, 0 g saturated fat, 0.1 g protein, 1 g carbohydrate, 0.1 g fiber, 4 mg sodium*

Easy Green Juice

Serves: 4 / Time: 5 minutes

INGREDIENTS

1 cup parsley

1 cup chopped celery

Juice of 1 lemon

½ inch fresh ginger, peeled

2 tablespoons organic apple cider vinegar

DIRECTIONS

Place all the ingredients in a high-speed blender and blend at high speed for 30 seconds.

Strain through a cheesecloth or a nut cloth.

Store in an airtight glass jar in the refrigerator for 3 to 4 days. If separation occurs, gently shake or stir it.

Nutrition information per serving: *15 calories, 0.2 g fat, 0 g saturated fat, 0.7 g protein, 2.9 g carbohydrate, 0.9 g fiber, 29 mg sodium*

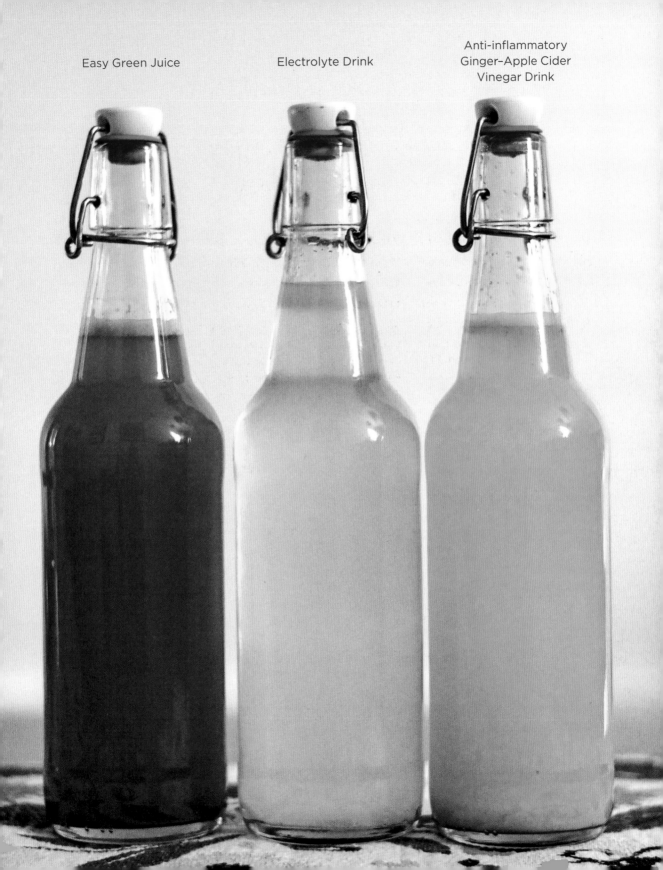

Easy Green Juice

Electrolyte Drink

Anti-inflammatory
Ginger–Apple Cider
Vinegar Drink

Electrolyte Drink

Serves: 3 / Time: 5 minutes

INGREDIENTS

1 cup filtered water

2 cups organic unsweetened coconut water

1 teaspoon sea salt

Juice of 1 lemon

5 to 10 drops liquid stevia

1 teaspoon magnesium powder (optional)

DIRECTIONS

Place all the ingredients in a glass jar and stir well.

Cover with an airtight lid and store in the refrigerator for up to 1 week.

Nutrition information per serving: *35 calories, 0.1 g fat, 0 g saturated fat, 0.1 g protein, 8.7 g carbohydrate, 0.1 g fiber, 179 mg sodium*

Apple Pie Smoothie

Serves: 1 / Time: 5 minutes

INGREDIENTS

½ **Granny Smith apple, cored**

¼ **cup almond butter**

½ **cup coconut cream**

½ **cup unsweetened almond milk**

½ **tablespoon Ceylon cinnamon**

¼ **teaspoon powdered ginger**

5 to 10 **drops liquid stevia**

1 **cup ice**

1 **ml CBD hemp oil (optional)**

DIRECTIONS

Place all the ingredients in a high-speed blender and blend until smooth.

Nutrition information per serving: *388 calories, 32.9 g fat, 25.6 g saturated fat, 4.6 g protein, 26.4 g carbohydrate, 8.1 g fiber, 95 mg sodium*

Blueberry Smoothie

Serves: 1 / Time: 5 minutes

INGREDIENTS

½ cup full-fat coconut milk

½ cup fresh baby spinach

½ cup frozen wild blueberries

1 scoop keto collagen powder

1 tablespoon almond butter

DIRECTIONS

Place all the ingredients in a high-speed blender and blend until smooth.

MAKE IT VEGAN

Omit the keto collagen powder and add 1 tablespoon coconut oil.

Nutrition information per serving: *454 calories, 36.2 g fat, 25.1 g saturated fat, 19.6 g protein, 16.2 g carbohydrate, 3.9 g fiber, 33 mg sodium*

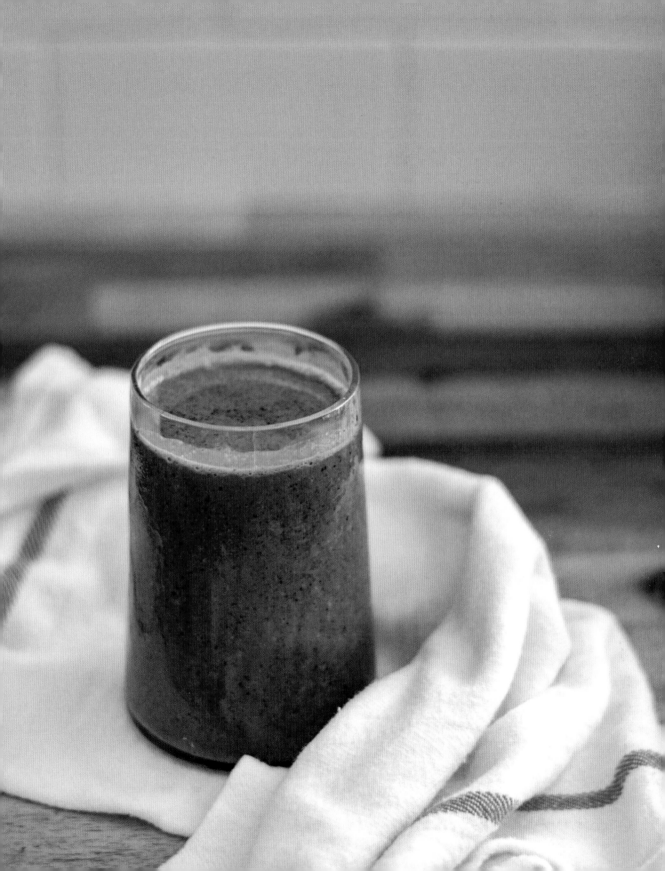

Matcha Green Tea Latte

Serves: 1 / Time: 5 minutes

INGREDIENTS

1½ cups almond or coconut milk

1 teaspoon ceremonial-grade matcha

1 scoop keto collagen powder

1 teaspoon coconut oil

2 teaspoons coconut butter

1 to 2 teaspoons maple syrup (optional)

Cinnamon, for topping

DIRECTIONS

Warm the milk in a tea kettle or small pot over low heat.

Pour the milk into a high-speed blender. Add the remaining ingredients, except the cinnamon.

Blend on high until well combined.

Top with cinnamon, and enjoy!

Nutrition information per serving: *320 calories, 25.3 g fat, 5.8 g saturated fat, 13.4 g protein, 14.3 g carbohydrate, 7.4 g fiber, 320 mg sodium*

Keto Coffee Shake

Serves: 2 / Time: 5 minutes

INGREDIENTS

1½ cups cold brew coffee

2 teaspoons MCT oil

½ cup almond milk

2 tablespoons
coconut cream

5 to 10 drops liquid stevia

1 cup ice

DIRECTIONS

Place all the ingredients in a high-speed blender and blend until smooth.

Nutrition information per serving: *243 calories, 22.1 g fat, 20.3 g saturated fat, 1.8 g protein, 13.4 g carbohydrate, 1.4 g fiber, 20 mg sodium*

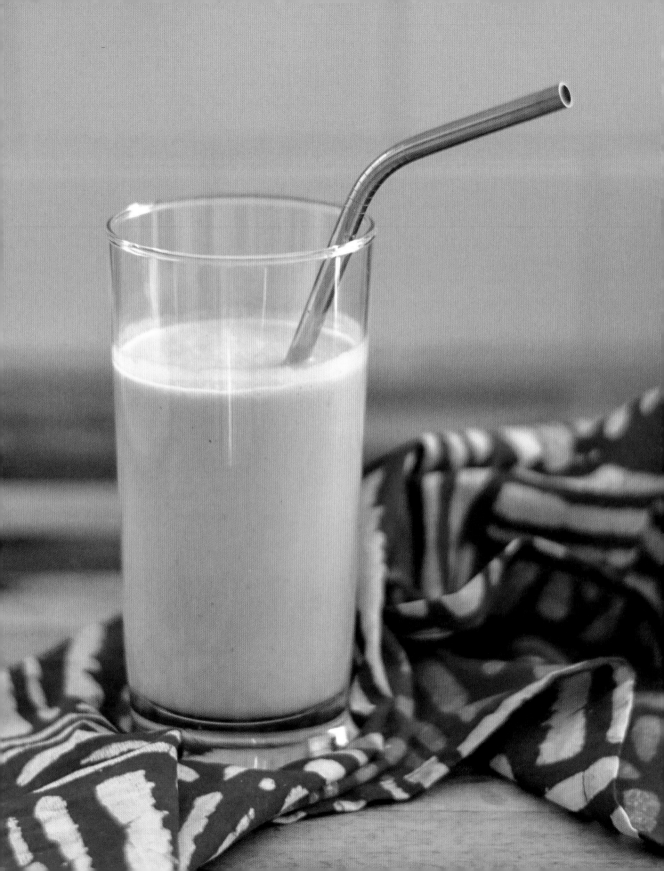

Keto Collagen Shake

Serves: 1 / Time: 5 minutes

INGREDIENTS

1 cup full-fat coconut milk

¼ cup cold water

1 scoop collagen protein

1 scoop vanilla bone broth protein

1 tablespoon goji berry powder

DIRECTIONS

Place all the ingredients in a high-speed blender and blend on low until smooth.

Nutrition information per serving: *601 calories, 49.2 g fat, 42.8 g saturated fat, 32.6 g protein, 13.4 g carbohydrate, 0 g fiber, 256 mg sodium*

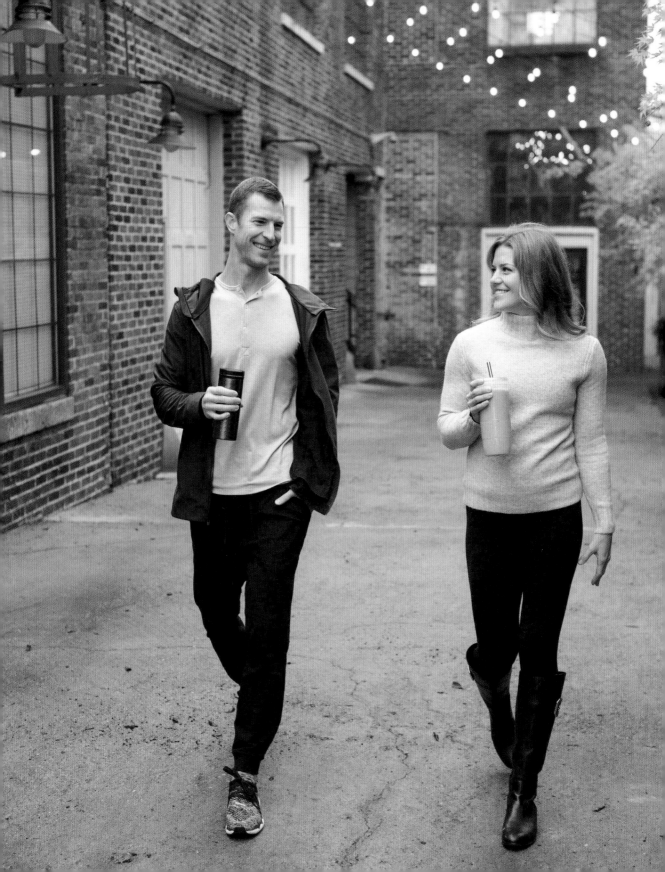

Strawberry Lemonade Slushy

Serves: 2 / Time: 5 minutes

INGREDIENTS

1 cup water

1 cup frozen strawberries

Juice of 1 lemon

5 to 10 drops liquid stevia

½ cup ice

2 scoops collagen protein (optional)

DIRECTIONS

Place all the ingredients in a high-speed blender and blend until a slushy consistency forms.

Nutrition information per serving: *60 calories, 0.1 g fat, 0 g saturated fat, 7.1 g protein, 8.6 g carbohydrate, 1.6 g fiber, 45 mg sodium*

Turmeric Golden Milk

Serves: 2 / Time: 10 minutes

INGREDIENTS

3 cups unsweetened almond milk

2 tablespoons coconut cream

2 teaspoons ground turmeric

1 teaspoon ground ginger

½ teaspoon freshly ground black pepper

2 cinnamon sticks (or 1 teaspoon ground cinnamon)

2 tablespoons coconut oil or ghee

5 to 6 drops liquid stevia

DIRECTIONS

Place the almond milk, coconut cream, turmeric, ginger, and black pepper in a high-speed blender. Pulse several times.

Pour the milk mixture into a small saucepan. Over medium heat, bring it to near boil. Reduce the heat to low at the first sign of boiling.

Stir in the cinnamon sticks, coconut oil, and stevia. Cover and let simmer for 5 minutes.

Discard the cinnamon sticks (if using), stir again, and serve immediately. Can be stored in the refrigerator for up to 2 days.

Nutrition information per serving: *268 calories, 22.7 g fat, 17 g saturated fat, 2.1 g protein, 16.5 g carbohydrate, 2.9 g fiber, 278 mg sodium*

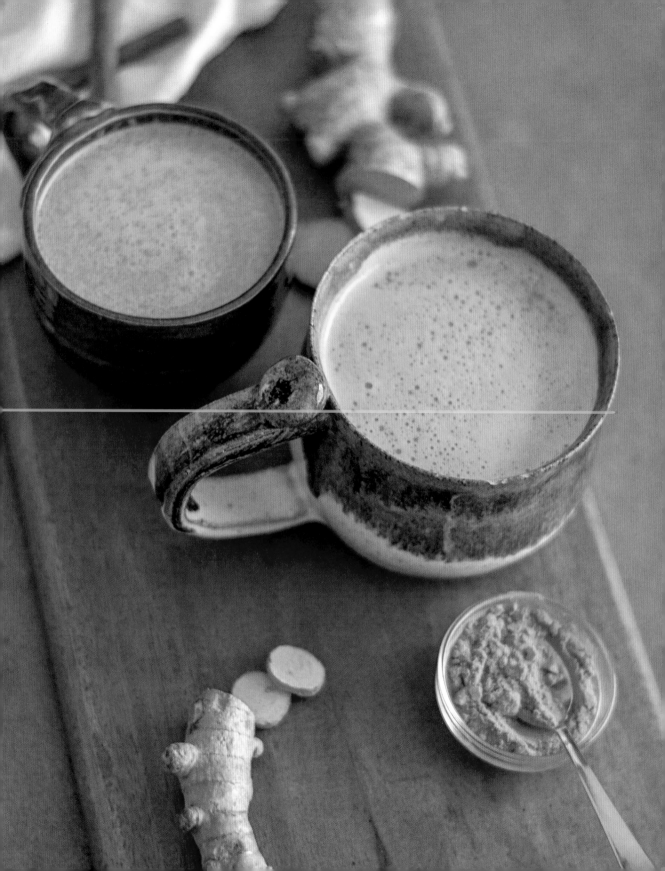

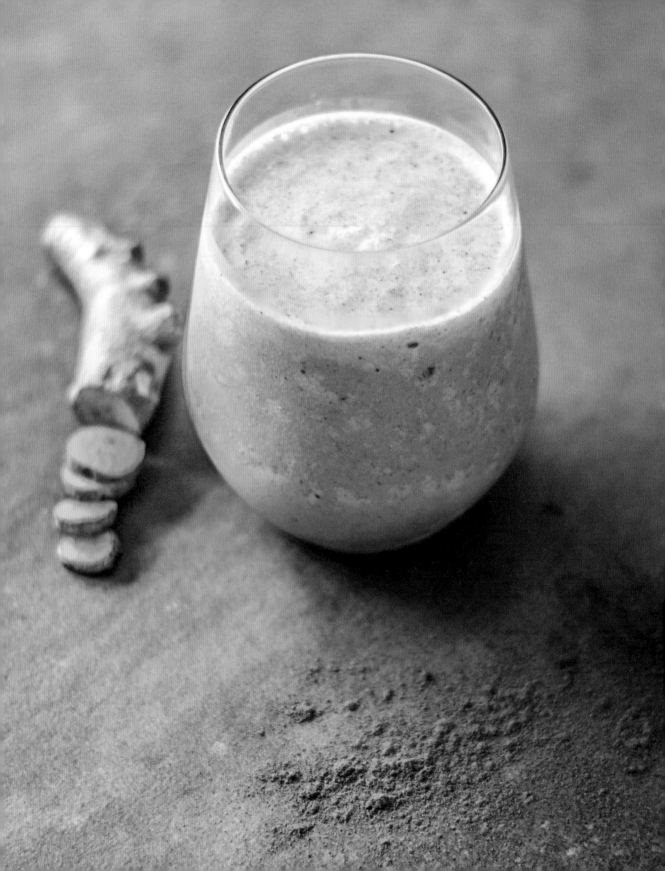

Turmeric Smoothie

Serves: 1 / Time: 5 minutes

INGREDIENTS

¾ cup full-fat coconut milk

¼ cup unsweetened
almond milk

1 teaspoon ground turmeric

½ teaspoon ground ginger

¼ teaspoon cinnamon

¼ teaspoon freshly ground
black pepper

1 scoop collagen protein

5 drops liquid stevia

5 to 6 ice cubes

½ avocado

DIRECTIONS

Place all the ingredients, except the ice cubes and avocado, in a high-speed blender. Pulse several times.

Add the ice cubes and avocado and blend at high speed until smooth.

MAKE IT VEGAN

Omit the collagen protein and add a plant-based keto protein powder.

Nutrition information per serving: *536 calories, 50.8 g fat, 33.7 g saturated fat, 11 g protein, 17.1 g carbohydrate, 7.3 g fiber, 113 mg sodium*

Smoothies and Drinks

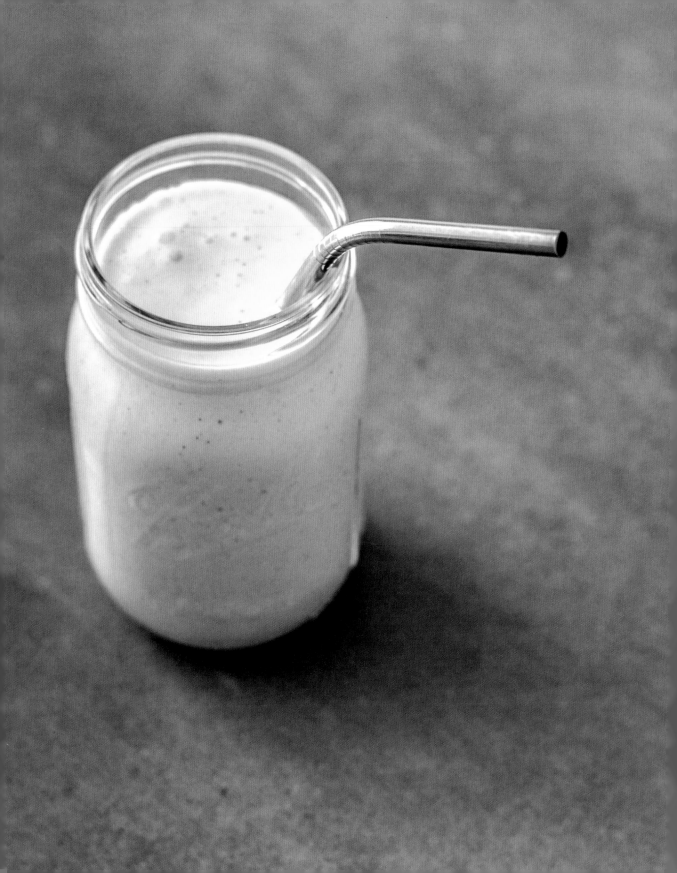

Vanilla Bean Smoothie

Serves: 1 / Time: 5 minutes

INGREDIENTS

1 cup full-fat coconut milk

½ teaspoon vanilla extract

1 scoop vanilla bone broth protein

½ cup water

1 cup ice

Pinch of sea salt

2 to 3 drops liquid stevia (optional)

DIRECTIONS

Place all the ingredients in a high-speed blender and blend until smooth.

Nutrition information per serving: *549 calories, 49.2 g fat, 42.8 g saturated fat, 24.6 g protein, 8.6 g carbohydrate, 0 g fiber, 417 mg sodium*

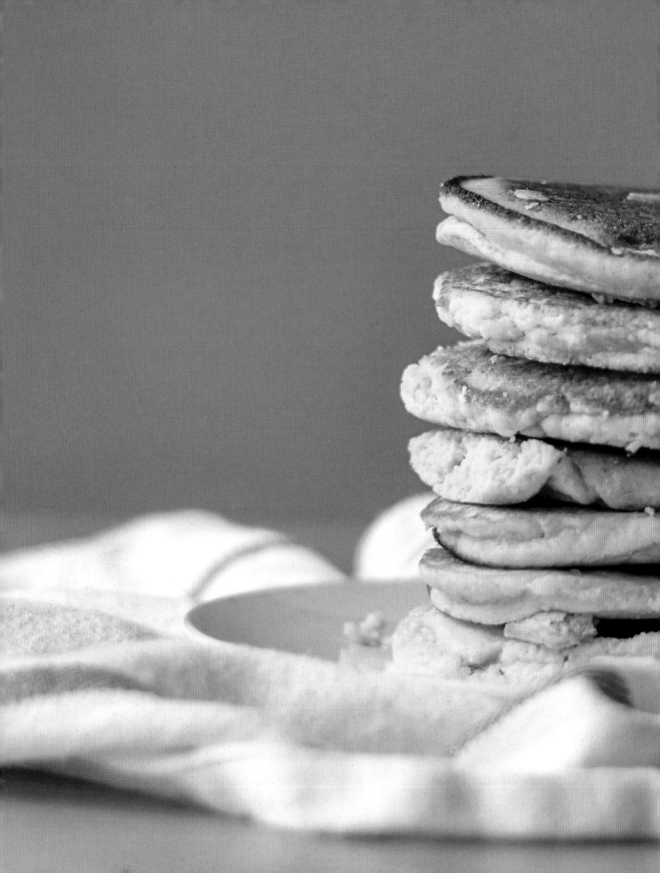

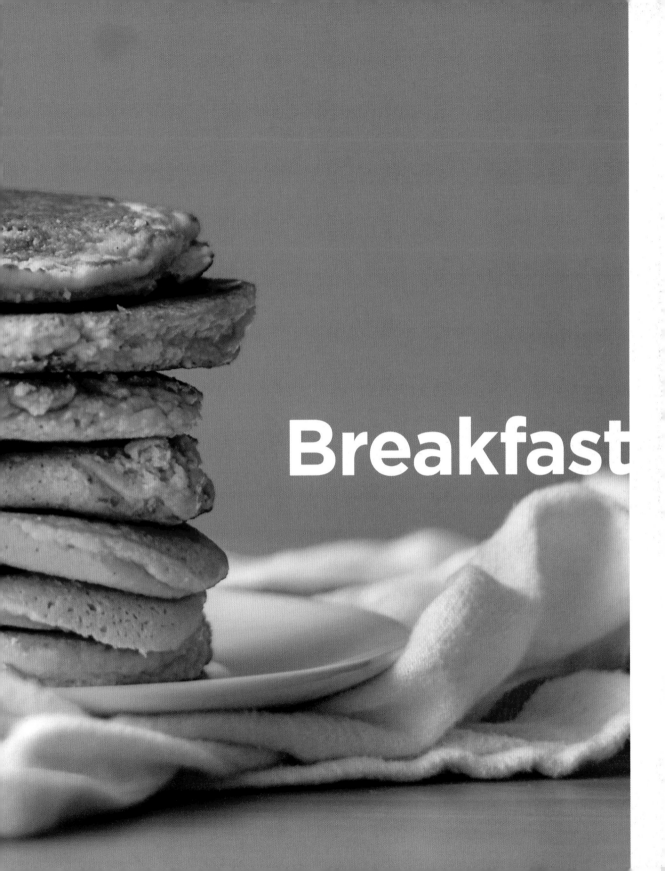

Breakfast

Baked Spinach Eggs

Serves: 4 / Time: 25 minutes

INGREDIENTS

2 tablespoons coconut oil

1 shallot, chopped

6 cups firmly packed spinach leaves

2 tablespoons chopped sun-dried tomatoes

4 large eggs

1 teaspoon Italian seasoning

Sea salt and freshly ground black pepper, to taste

1 ounce raw cheddar cheese, grated

DIRECTIONS

Preheat the oven to 400°F.

Heat the coconut oil in a skillet over medium heat.

Add the shallot and cook for two minutes.

Add the spinach and cook for 3 to 4 minutes, stirring occasionally.

Add the sun-dried tomatoes and mix well. Distribute the spinach/tomato mixture into four ramekins.

Crack one egg into each ramekin over the spinach mixture. Sprinkle the Italian seasoning, salt, and pepper over each egg.

Place the ramekins on a baking sheet and bake for 15 to 18 minutes. Remove from the oven and sprinkle the cheddar on top.

Nutrition information per serving: *195 calories, 15.1 g fat, 9 g saturated fat, 11.6 g protein, 8.4 g carbohydrate, 3.5 g fiber, 367 mg sodium*

Salmon Egg Bake

Serves: 4 / Time: 55 minutes

INGREDIENTS

2 tablespoons ghee

1 medium onion, thinly sliced crosswise

1 cup of combined red, yellow, and orange peppers, chopped

1 cup chopped mushrooms

6 ounces smoked wild-caught Alaskan salmon, skin removed and salmon cut into 1-inch pieces

8 large eggs

1 cup plain kefir

1 tablespoon chopped fresh dill

¼ teaspoon sea salt

¼ teaspoon freshly ground black pepper

1 teaspoon nutmeg

¾ cup goat cheese (chèvre), crumbled

DIRECTIONS

Preheat the oven to 350°F. Grease a baking pan with coconut oil.

Melt the ghee in a 10-inch skillet over medium-high heat. Add the onion and peppers and cook, stirring occasionally, for 3 minutes, or until soft and translucent.

Add the mushrooms and cook for 3 to 4 minutes, or until softened and slightly browned. Remove the skillet from the heat.

Spread the onion mixture over the bottom of the prepared baking pan.

Spread the salmon pieces over the onion mixture.

Beat the eggs in a medium bowl with the kefir, dill, salt, pepper, and nutmeg.

Pour the egg mixture over the onion mixture.

Bake for 35 to 40 minutes.

Sprinkle the goat cheese on top and serve.

Nutrition information per serving: *772 calories, 51.2 g fat, 29.3 g saturated fat, 65.8 g protein, 12.5 g carbohydrate, 2.1 g fiber, 576 mg sodium*

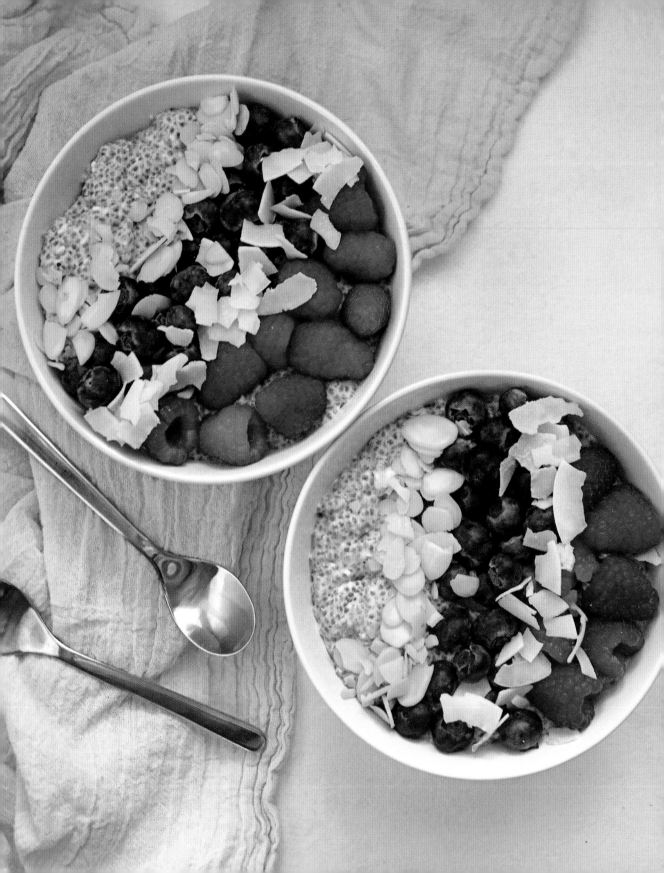

Chia Pudding Bowls

Serves: 2 / Time: 35 minutes

INGREDIENTS

Pudding:

1 cup full-fat coconut milk

1 cup unsweetened
almond milk

1 teaspoon vanilla extract

½ cup chia seeds

5 to 10 drops liquid stevia

Toppings:

¼ cup blueberries

¼ cup raspberries

¼ cup sliced almonds

¼ cup coconut flakes

DIRECTIONS

In a medium bowl, combine all the pudding ingredients and stir together. Refrigerate for at least 30 minutes or overnight.

When the pudding has thickened, divide into two bowls, add the toppings, and serve.

Nutrition information per serving: *449 calories, 29.2 g fat, 8.9 g saturated fat, 16.2 g protein, 30.3 g carbohydrate, 24.3 g fiber, 85 mg sodium*

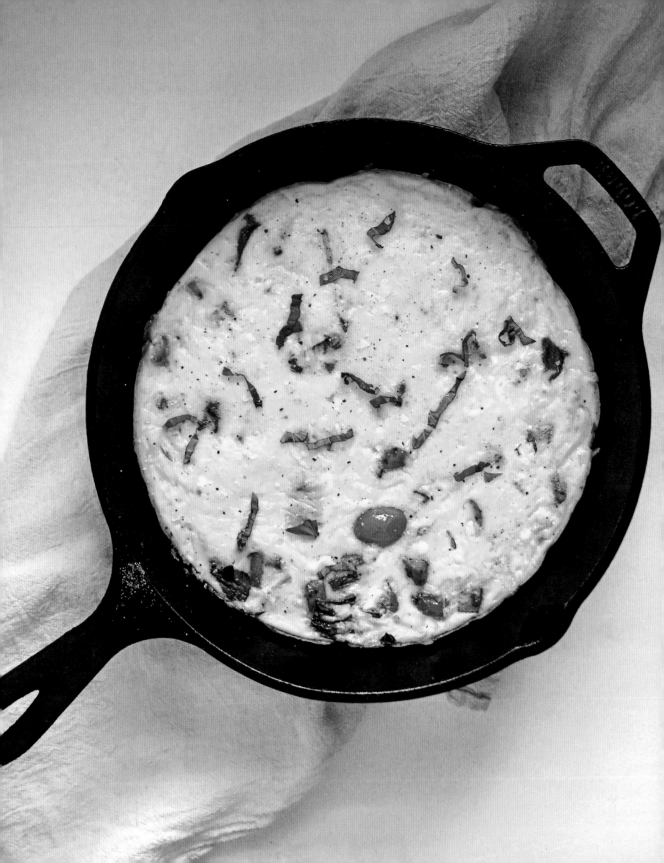

Frittata

Serves: 6 / Time: 30 minutes

INGREDIENTS

2 links organic chicken sausage (with no added sugar), diced

1 cup fresh spinach

½ cup asparagus, chopped

6 large eggs

2 tablespoons unsweetened almond milk

½ cup cherry tomatoes, sliced in half

1 cup shredded, organic mozzarella cheese

DIRECTIONS

Preheat the oven to 375°F.

Brown the chicken sausage in a cast-iron skillet or oven-proof pan.

Add the spinach and asparagus to the skillet and cook for 2 minutes, or until the spinach has wilted.

Whisk together the eggs and almond milk. Stir in the tomatoes.

Pour the egg mixture into the skillet and bake the fritatta for 20 to 22 minutes, or until the eggs are cooked through.

Remove the frittata and sprinkle with the mozzarella. Cut into wedges and serve. Store in an airtight container in the refrigerator for up to 4 days.

MAKE IT VEGETARIAN
Omit the chicken sausage.

MAKE IT DAIRY FREE
Omit the cheese or use a dairy-free cheese.

Nutrition information per serving: *134 calories, 7.3 g fat, 2.7 g saturated fat, 13.2 g protein, 4.7 g carbohydrate, 0.9 g fiber, 273 mg sodium*

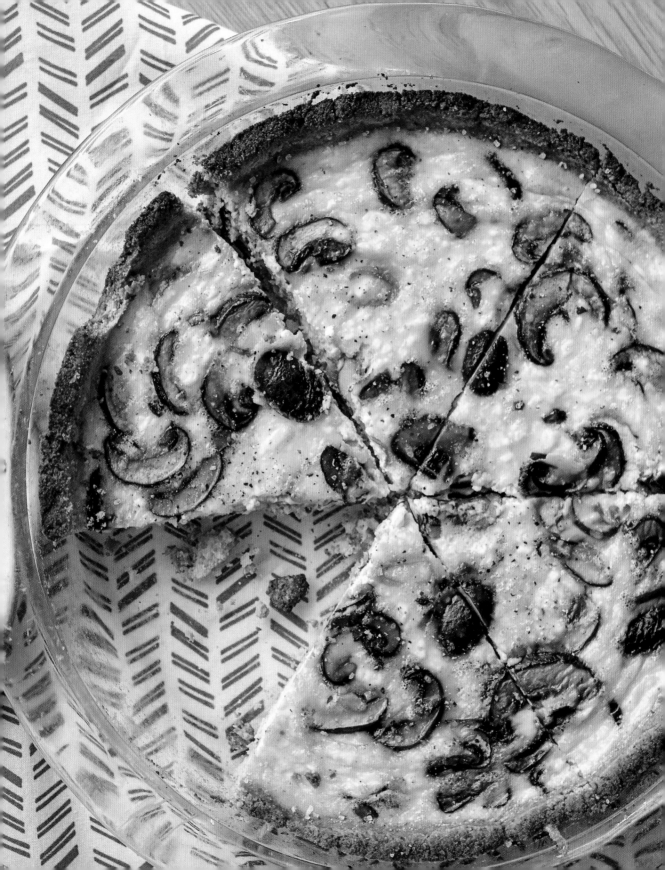

Grain-Free Quiche

Serves: 8 / Time: 1 hour

INGREDIENTS

Crust:

1¾ cups almond flour

¼ cup coconut flour

1 garlic clove, minced

1 teaspoon dried oregano

Pinch of sea salt

⅓ cup avocado or extra virgin olive oil

2 tablespoons water

Filling:

1 tablespoon avocado or extra virgin olive oil

2 garlic cloves, minced

1 cup cremini or button mushrooms, thinly sliced

½ shallot, sliced

6 large eggs

⅓ cup unsweetened almond milk

½ teaspoon sea salt

2 ounces goat cheese (chèvre), crumbled

DIRECTIONS

Preheat the oven to 400°F. Grease a 9-inch pie pan.

In a medium bowl, combine all the crust ingredients. Mix well until the dough has a crumbly texture.

Place the dough in the pie pan and, with clean hands, press it out evenly over the bottom and 1 to 1¼ inches up the sides of the pan.

Bake for 15 minutes.

Meanwhile, in a medium skillet over medium heat, heat the avocado oil. Sauté the garlic, mushrooms, and shallot for 5 minutes. Set aside to cool.

In a large bowl, beat the eggs and almond milk. Add the salt and gently stir in the vegetable mixture and goat cheese.

Pour the filling into the baked crust, reduce the oven temperature to 375°F, and bake for 30 minutes, or until the eggs are cooked through.

Cut in wedges and serve. Leftovers can be stored in the refrigerator for up to 2 days.

MAKE IT DAIRY FREE

Use an alternative plant-based goat "cheese," or omit the cheese altogether.

GIVE IT A COLLAGEN BOOST

Add 1 scoop of collagen protein to the beaten eggs before adding the vegetable mixture.

Nutrition information per serving: *463 calories, 37.4 g fat, 5.9 g saturated fat, 20.8 g protein, 19 g carbohydrate, 9.7 g fiber, 198 mg sodium*

Heart-Healthy Eggs Benedict with Asparagus

Serves: 2 / Time: 20 minutes

INGREDIENTS

1 to 2 teaspoons coconut or avocado oil

1 bunch asparagus (16 stalks)

2 to 3 cups water, plus ½ tablespoon

2 large eggs

2 tablespoons grass-fed butter or ghee

¼ teaspoon Dijon mustard

1 tablespoon lemon juice

¼ teaspoon sea salt

¼ tomato, sliced

½ avocado, sliced

Chives, chopped, for topping

DIRECTIONS

In a medium frying pan, heat the coconut oil over medium heat.

Add the asparagus and sauté for 8 to 10 minutes, or until fork-tender.

In a small pot, bring the 2 to 3 cups water to a boil.

Gently lower the eggs into the water and cook for 5 minutes. Remove the eggs and set aside.

In a small saucepan, melt the butter or ghee over medium-low heat. Peel the eggs.

Place the melted butter, eggs, Dijon mustard, lemon juice, salt, and the remaining ½ tablespoon water in a high-speed blender and blend until well combined. Let the sauce sit to combine the flavors.

Divide the asparagus between two plates and top with the tomato and avocado.

Drizzle the egg sauce over the asparagus.

Top with the chives and serve.

Nutrition information per serving: *340 calories, 30 g fat, 12.8 g saturated fat, 10.9 g protein, 10.7 g carbohydrate, 6.4 g fiber, 315 mg sodium*

Huevos Rancheros

Serves: 6 / Time: 25 minutes

INGREDIENTS

2 tablespoons coconut oil

½ pound grass-fed ground beef

½ red onion, diced

1 small jalapeño, stem removed, diced (seeds removed, optional)

2 tablespoons grass-fed cream cheese

1 teaspoon dried oregano

Sea salt and freshly ground pepper to taste

4 to 6 large eggs, fried or scrambled

Paleo tortillas or bibb lettuce

Toppings:

1 to 2 tomatoes, diced

1 avocado, pitted and diced

Fresh cilantro, chopped

DIRECTIONS

Place the coconut oil and beef in a large skillet over medium heat. Cook, stirring occasionally, for 5 to 7 minutes, or until the beef is browned.

Add the onion, jalapeño, cream cheese, oregano, salt, and pepper, stirring until the onion becomes translucent. Remove from the heat.

Cook the eggs in another pan over medium-low heat.

Place the Paleo tortillas on six plates, top with the meat mixture and eggs, and add the tomato, avocado, and cilantro toppings to serve.

Nutrition information per serving: *298 calories, 21.8 g fat, 7.9 g saturated fat, 17.5 g protein, 9.8 g carbohydrate, 2.9 g fiber, 231 mg sodium*

Breakfast

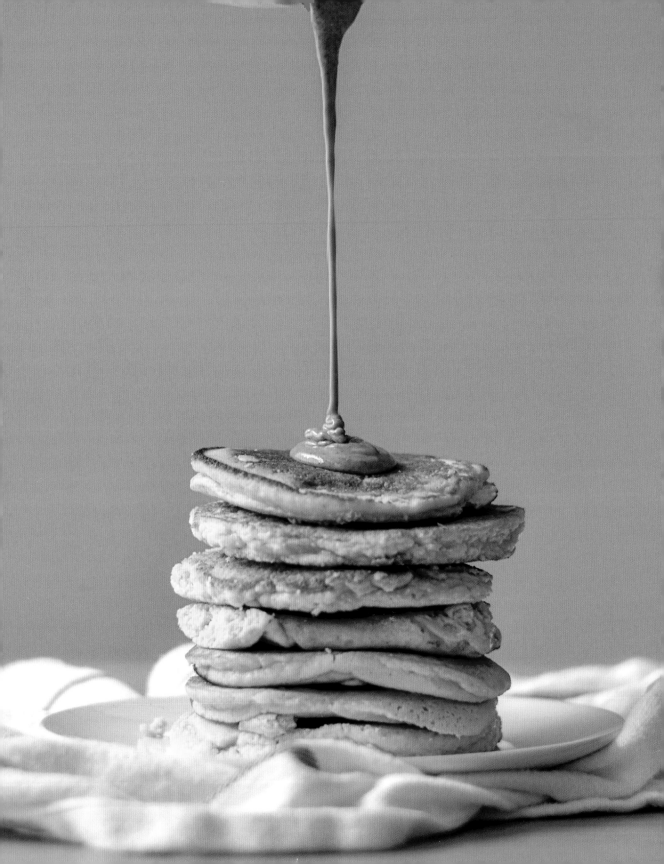

Keto Pancakes

Serves: 5 (2 pancakes per serving) / Time: 20 minutes

INGREDIENTS

¾ cup almond flour

¼ cup coconut flour

1 scoop vanilla bone broth protein or keto collagen powder

1 teaspoon baking powder

¼ teaspoon sea salt

3 large eggs

¼ cup coconut cream

1 teaspoon monk fruit sweetener

3 tablespoons water

1 tablespoon coconut oil, melted

¼ cup almond butter (optional)

DIRECTIONS

In a large bowl, mix together the almond flour, coconut flour, bone broth protein, baking powder, and salt. Set aside.

In a medium bowl, beat together the eggs, coconut cream, and monk fruit sweetener with a fork or whisk. Beat for 30 seconds, or until very fluffy.

Incorporate the egg mixture into the flour mixture, stirring well. Add the water and coconut oil and stir until it forms a thick batter.

In a large greased skillet over medium heat, add the batter by the spoonful.

Cook for 3 to 4 minutes. Flip the pancakes when they lift easily off the skillet with a spatula and cook on the other side for 2 to 3 minutes.

Melt the almond butter (if using). Serve the pancakes with the almond butter poured over the top.

MAKE IT VEGAN

Replace the eggs with 3 tablespoons flaxseed powder and ½ cup water.

Omit the bone broth protein or keto collagen powder.

Add 2 more tablespoons water and 1 more tablespoon coconut oil.

Nutrition information per serving: *203 calories, 14.5 g fat, 7.9 g saturated fat, 11.8 g protein, 8.5 g carbohydrate, 4 g fiber, 204 mg sodium*

Keto Waffles

Serves: 1 / Time: 10 minutes

INGREDIENTS

2 large eggs

1 tablespoon unsweetened, vanilla-flavored almond milk

1 teaspoon vanilla extract

1 scoop vanilla keto protein powder

1 teaspoon baking powder

Pinch of sea salt

1 tablespoon butter

½ teaspoon cinnamon

DIRECTIONS

Preheat a waffle maker and spray with nonstick spray.

In a mixing bowl, whisk together the eggs, almond milk, and vanilla extract until bubbly.

Add the protein powder, baking powder, and salt to the wet ingredients and whisk until combined.

Pour ¼ cup of the batter into the waffle maker and cook until golden brown. Remove to a plate. Continue making waffles until the batter is used up.

Spread the waffles with butter and sprinkle with cinnamon.

Nutrition information per serving: *437 calories, 32.7 g fat, 15.4 g saturated fat, 27.8 g protein, 6.7 g carbohydrate, 0.8 g fiber, 612 mg sodium*

Low-Carb Egg Muffins

Serves: 6 / Time: 20 minutes

INGREDIENTS

6 large eggs

¼ cup unsweetened almond milk

¼ cup freshly grated Parmesan cheese

Sea salt and freshly ground black pepper, to taste

DIRECTIONS

Preheat the oven to 375°F. Grease a 6-cup muffin mold or line with paper cups.

In a medium bowl, beat together the eggs and almond milk.

Divide the egg mixture evenly among the prepared muffin cups, filling each cup about three-quarters full.

Top with the Parmesan, salt, and pepper. Bake for 15 minutes or until the eggs are cooked through, and serve immediately.

MAKE IT DAIRY FREE
Omit the Parmesan or use a dairy-free cheese.

GIVE IT A COLLAGEN BOOST
Add 1 scoop of collagen protein to the egg mixture.

Nutrition information per serving: *78 calories, 5.4 g fat, 2 g saturated fat, 6.9 g protein, 0.6 g carbohydrate, 0.1 g fiber, 146 mg sodium*

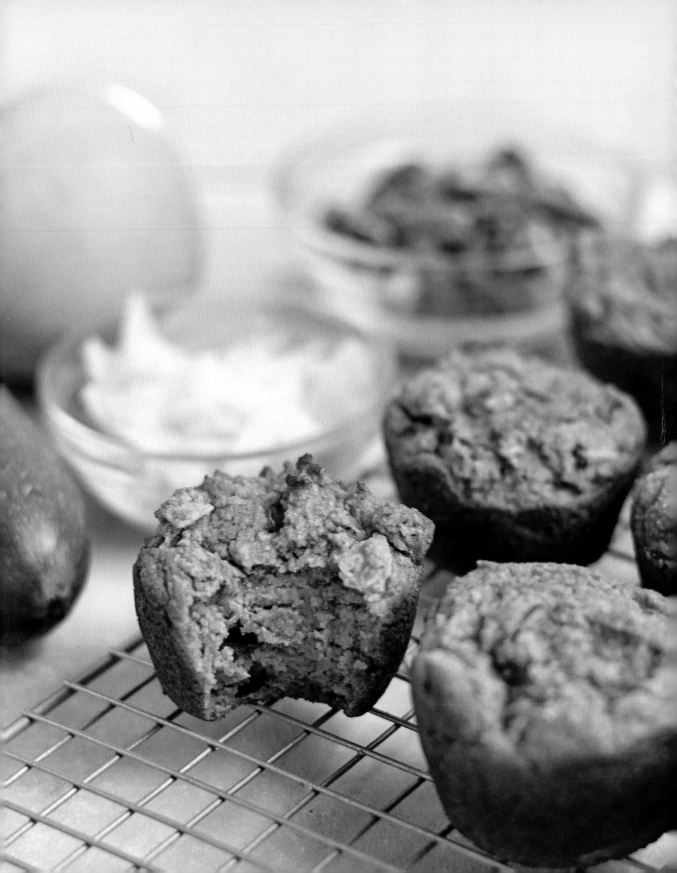

Morning Glory
Keto Muffins

Serves: 12 / Time: 35 minutes

INGREDIENTS

2 cups almond flour

1 teaspoon baking powder

1 teaspoon baking soda

½ teaspoon sea salt

2 teaspoons cinnamon

2 scoops keto collagen powder (optional)

1 cup pumpkin purée

2 large pasture-raised eggs

¼ cup all-natural almond butter

¼ cup monk fruit syrup, maple flavored

1 apple, cored and shredded

1 small zucchini, shredded

½ cup chopped pecans

½ cup coconut flakes

DIRECTIONS

Preheat the oven to 375°F. Grease a 12-cup muffin mold or line with paper cups.

In a medium bowl, mix the almond flour, baking powder, baking soda, sea salt, cinnamon, and keto collagen powder (if using) together and set aside.

In a large bowl, mix the pumpkin purée, eggs, almond butter, and monk fruit syrup together. Stir in the dry ingredients and combine well.

Gently fold in the apple, zucchini, pecans, and coconut flakes.

Divide the mixture evenly among the prepared muffin cups.

Bake for 22 to 24 minutes, or until a toothpick comes out clean when inserted in the center.

Store the muffins in an airtight container at room temperature for up to 3 days, or freeze them for longer storage.

Nutrition information per serving: *258 calories, 20.8 g fat, 3.3 g saturated fat, 10.7 g protein, 9.1 g carbohydrate, 5.4 g fiber, 180 mg sodium*

Collagen-Boosting Blueberry Muffins

Serves: 12 / Time: 35 minutes

INGREDIENTS

2 cups almond flour

½ cup coconut flour

1½ teaspoons baking powder

¼ teaspoon sea salt

2 scoops keto collagen powder

⅓ cup full-fat coconut milk

3 large eggs

¼ cup monk fruit sweetener

3 tablespoons coconut oil, melted

¾ cup blueberries

DIRECTIONS

Preheat the oven to 350°F.

Grease a 12-cup muffin mold or line with paper cups.

In a large bowl, mix together the almond and coconut flours, baking powder, sea salt, and keto collagen powder. Set aside.

In a medium bowl, whisk together the coconut milk, eggs, monk fruit sweetener, and coconut oil.

Slowly add the milk mixture to the flour mixture, mixing constantly.

Fold in the blueberries and divide the mixture evenly into the muffin cups.

Bake for 20 minutes. Remove from the pan and let cool.

Store the muffins in an airtight container at room temperature for up to 3 days, or freeze them for longer storage.

MAKE IT VEGAN
Replace the eggs with 3 tablespoons flaxseed powder plus ½ cup water, and omit the keto collagen powder.

Nutrition information per serving: *134 calories, 8.9 g fat, 5.7 g saturated fat, 4.8 g protein, 11.5 g carbohydrate, 4.9 g fiber, 42 mg sodium*

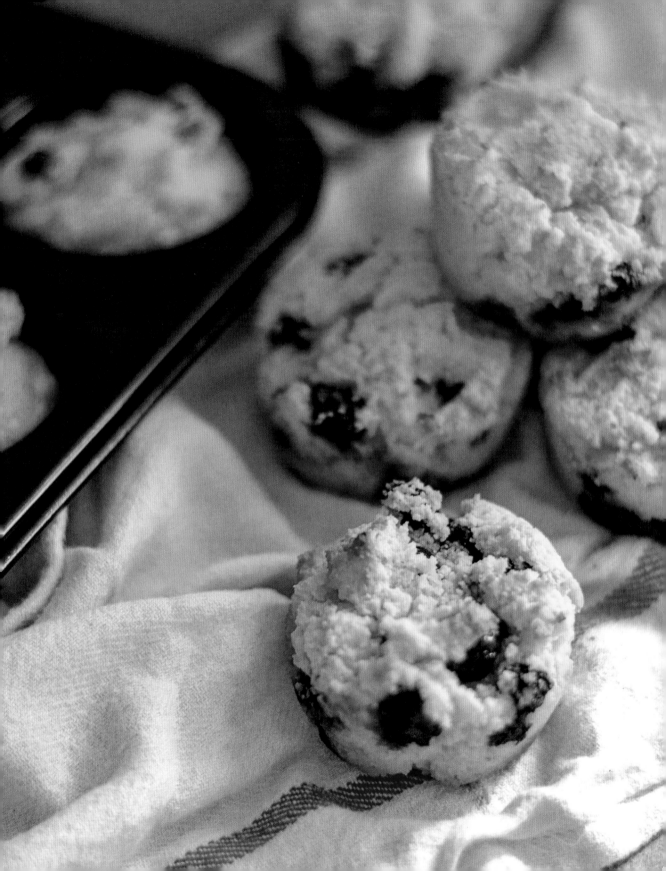

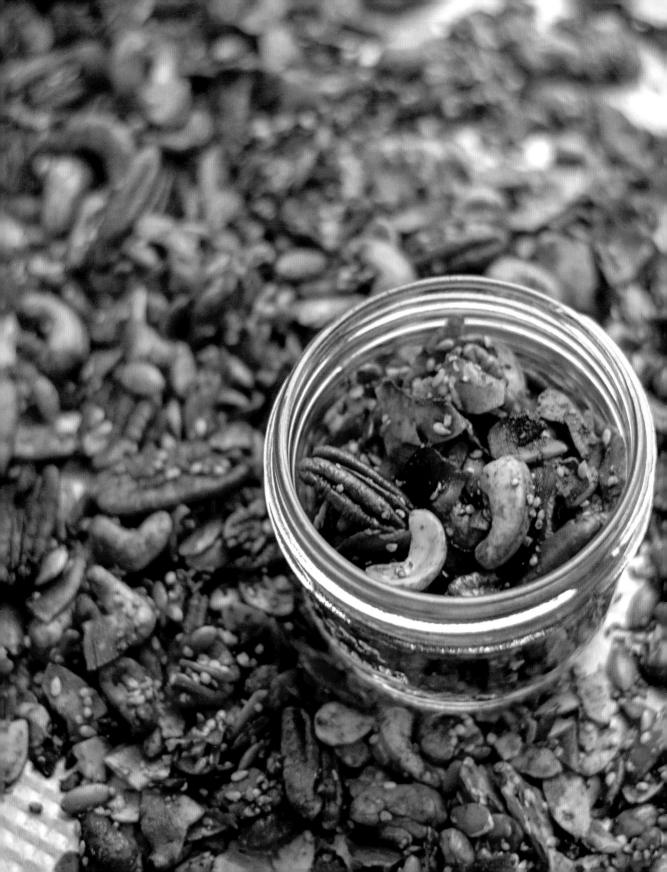

Granola

Serves: 6 / Time: 35 minutes

INGREDIENTS

½ cup unsweetened shredded coconut

1 cup raw almonds, slivered or sliced

1 cup raw walnuts or cashews

1 cup raw pecans

½ cup raw pumpkin seeds

¼ cup hemp seeds

1 cup cacao nibs

1 teaspoon cinnamon or pumpkin pie spice

¼ teaspoon sea salt

¼ cup coconut oil, melted

2 tablespoons monk fruit syrup, maple flavored

DIRECTIONS

Preheat the oven to 325°F. Line a baking sheet with parchment paper.

In a large bowl, mix together all the ingredients except the coconut oil and monk fruit syrup.

In a large saucepan over medium-low heat, stir the coconut oil and monk fruit syrup together until warm. Add all the other ingredients and mix well.

Spread the mixture evenly over the parchment-lined baking sheet.

Bake for 20 minutes.

Remove from the oven and stir the granola with a spatula. Return to the oven and bake for 5 minutes, or until golden brown.

Store in a glass container at room temperature. Consume within 3 weeks.

Nutrition information per serving: *649 calories, 53.9 g fat, 24 g saturated fat, 16.7 g protein, 28.7 g carbohydrate, 13.5 g fiber, 92 mg sodium*

Beef Bacon Quiche

Serves: 8 / Time: 50 minutes

INGREDIENTS

Crust:

1¾ cups almond flour

¼ cup coconut flour

1 garlic clove, minced

1 teaspoon dried oregano

Pinch of sea salt

⅓ cup avocado or extra virgin olive oil

2 tablespoons water

Filling:

1 to 2 tablespoons avocado oil

½ yellow onion, diced

1 red bell pepper, diced

1 small zucchini, diced

2 garlic cloves, minced

6 large pasture-raised eggs

4 slices organic beef bacon, cooked and chopped

1 cup shredded mozzarella cheese

DIRECTIONS

Preheat the oven to 400°F. Grease a 9-inch pie pan or quiche pan.

In a medium bowl, mix all the crust ingredients well. The dough will be crumbly.

Place the dough in the pie pan, and with clean hands, press it evenly over the bottom and 1 to 1¼ inches up the sides of the pan.

Bake the crust for 15 minutes.

Meanwhile, heat the avocado oil in a skillet over medium heat. Add the onion, bell pepper, zucchini, and garlic, and sauté for 5 to 7 minutes, or until the vegetables are soft.

Whisk the eggs in a mixing bowl and stir in the vegetables and bacon.

Pour the mixture into the crust, top with the cheese, and bake for 30 minutes, or until the eggs are cooked through.

Cut into wedges and serve.

MAKE IT DAIRY FREE

Omit the cheese or use a dairy-free cheese.

Nutrition information per serving: *328 calories, 24.2 g fat, 5.1 g saturated fat, 17.6 g protein, 15.2 g carbohydrate, 7.1 g fiber, 338 mg sodium*

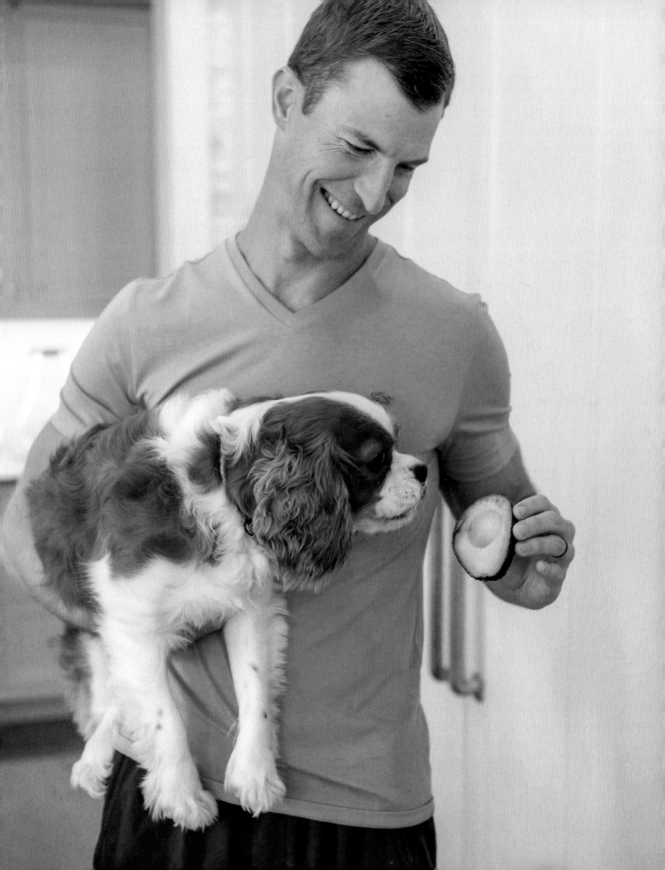

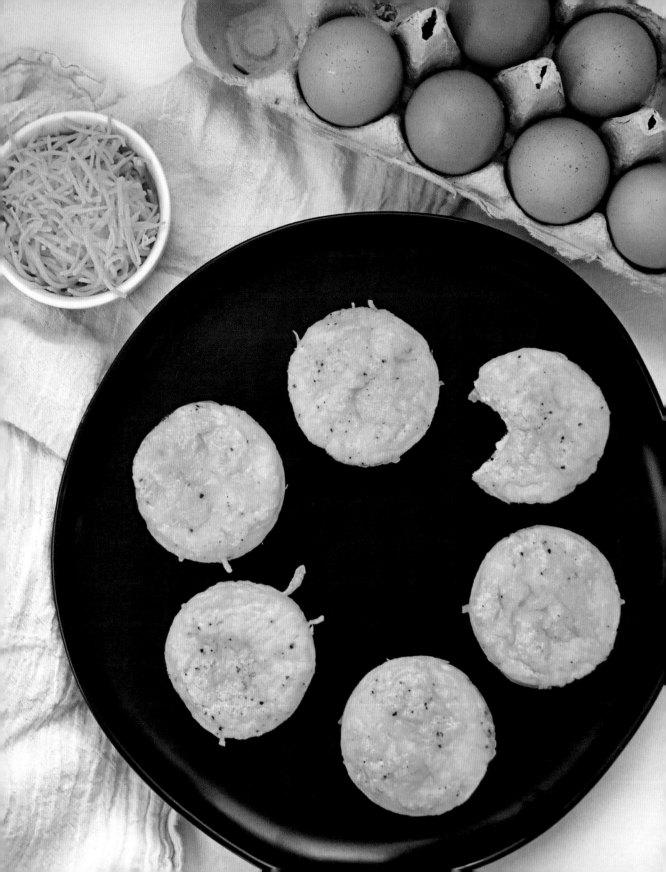

Turkey and Cheese Egg Bites

Makes: 6 / Time: 35 minutes

INGREDIENTS

6 large pasture-raised eggs

¼ cup unsweetened almond milk

Pinch of sea salt and freshly ground black pepper

½ cup shredded cheddar cheese

2 slices (about ½ cup) pasture-raised organic turkey, diced

DIRECTIONS

Preheat the oven to 350°F. Grease a 6-cup muffin mold or line with paper cups.

In a medium mixing bowl, whisk together the eggs, almond milk, salt, and pepper.

Divide the egg mixture evenly among the prepared muffin cups, filling each about three-quarters full.

Add the cheese and turkey slices equally among the muffin cups.

Bake for 25 to 30 minutes, or until the eggs are cooked through. Serve immediately.

MAKE IT DAIRY FREE
Omit the cheese or use a dairy-free cheese.

Nutrition information per serving: *116 calories, 7.3 g fat, 3.5 g saturated fat, 12.4 g protein, 1.2 g carbohydrate, 0.1 g fiber, 294 mg sodium*

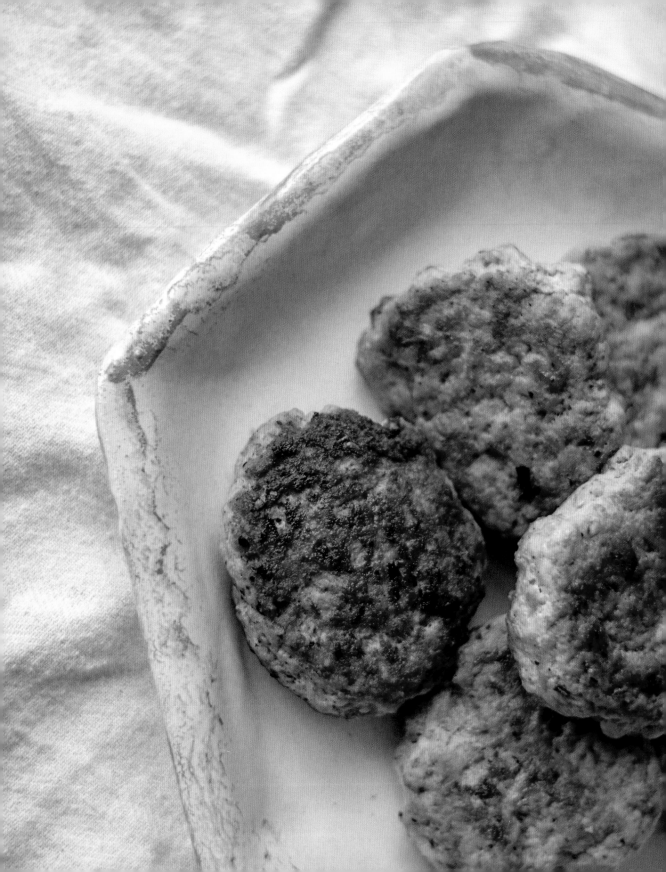

Turkey Breakfast Sausage

Serves: 4 (2 patties per serving) / Time: 15 minutes

INGREDIENTS

2 teaspoons dried sage

2 teaspoons sea salt

½ teaspoon freshly ground black pepper

½ teaspoon red pepper flakes

¼ teaspoon garlic powder

1 pound ground turkey

1 tablespoon avocado oil

DIRECTIONS

In a bowl, mix the spices and the ground turkey together with your hands until well combined.

Heat the avocado oil in a medium or large skillet over medium heat.

Form the meat mixture into 8 flat, round patties and carefully put them in the skillet with a spatula.

Cook each patty for 3 to 4 minutes on each side, or until cooked through. Serve immediately.

Nutrition information per serving: *229 calories, 13 g fat, 2.2 g saturated fat, 31.2 g protein, 0.8 g carbohydrate, 0.4 g fiber, 1058 mg sodium*

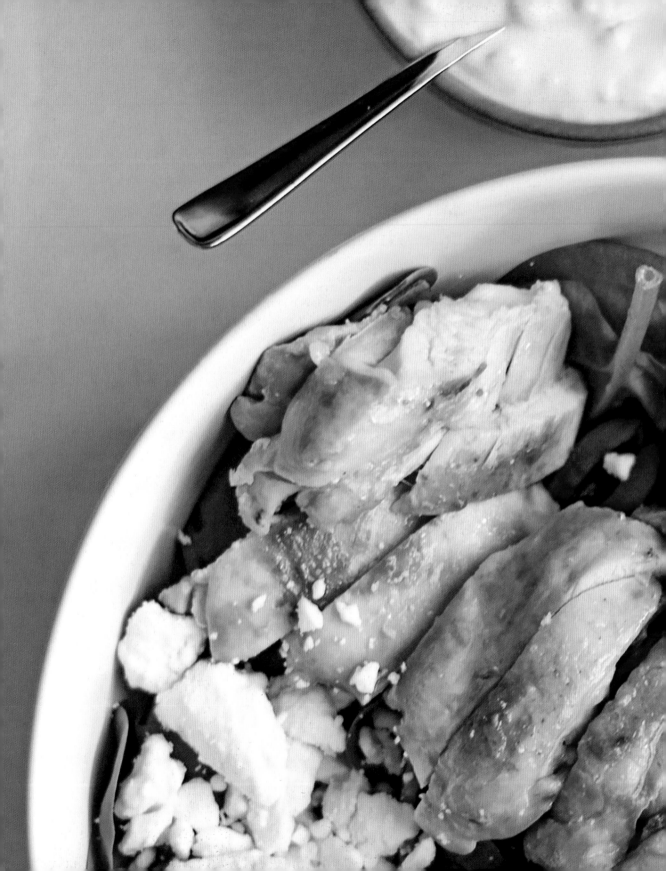

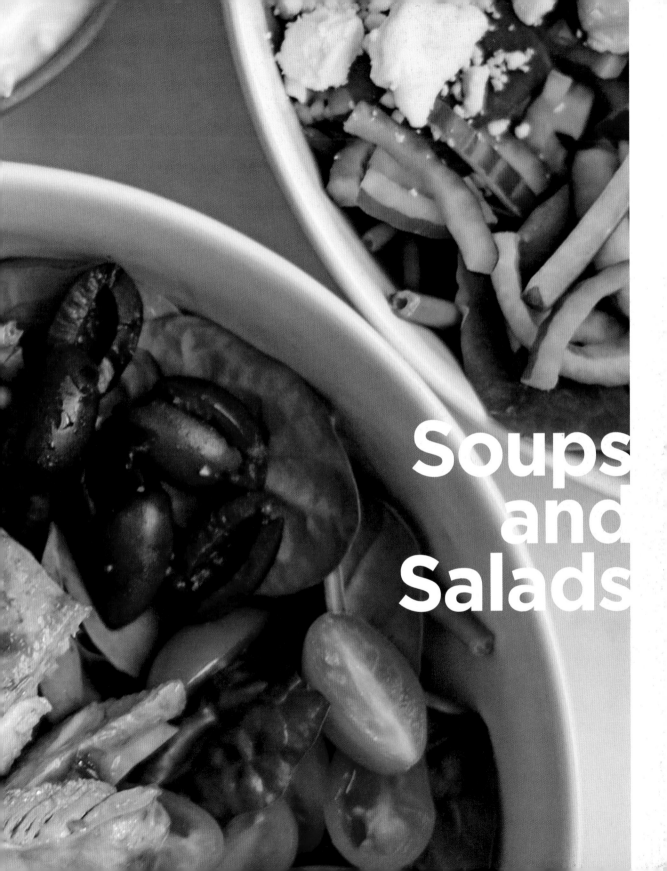

Soups
and
Salads

Albacore Tuna Salad

Serves: 4 / Time: 5 minutes

INGREDIENTS

2 (5-ounce) cans albacore tuna packed in water, drained

¼ cup avocado oil mayonnaise

2 teaspoons Dijon mustard

3 teaspoons dried dill

2 teaspoons lime juice

½ cup diced bell pepper

Mixed greens

DIRECTIONS

In a small bowl, combine the tuna, mayonnaise, mustard, dill, lime juice, and bell pepper.

Serve on a bed of mixed greens.

GIVE IT A COLLAGEN BOOST

Add 1 scoop of collagen protein.

Nutrition information per serving: *294 calories, 20.9 g fat, 3.1 g saturated fat, 13.4 g protein, 18.9 g carbohydrate, 7.4 g fiber, 313 mg sodium*

Cauliflower "Potato" Salad

Serves: 6 / Time: 1 hour, 30 minutes

INGREDIENTS

1 large cauliflower

Sea salt and freshly ground black pepper, to taste

3 hard-boiled eggs, diced

¾ cup avocado oil mayonnaise

2 tablespoons Dijon mustard

¼ cup dill pickle, diced

3 celery stalks, diced

1 tablespoon apple cider vinegar

1 teaspoon garlic powder

DIRECTIONS

Remove the stem and cut the cauliflower into florets.

Put 1 to 2 inches water in a large pot, add a pinch of salt, and bring to a boil. Add the cauliflower, reduce the heat to low, and cover the pot. Steam the cauliflower for 10 minutes, or until fork-tender.

Drain the cauliflower and let it cool for 15 minutes.

Mix the remaining ingredients in a large bowl. When cooled, add the cauliflower and mix together.

Cover and refrigerate for 1 to 2 hours, until chilled. Serve cold.

Nutrition information per serving: *305 calories, 29.8 g fat, 4.6 g saturated fat, 5.5 g protein, 3.6 g carbohydrate, 1.4 g fiber, 573 mg sodium*

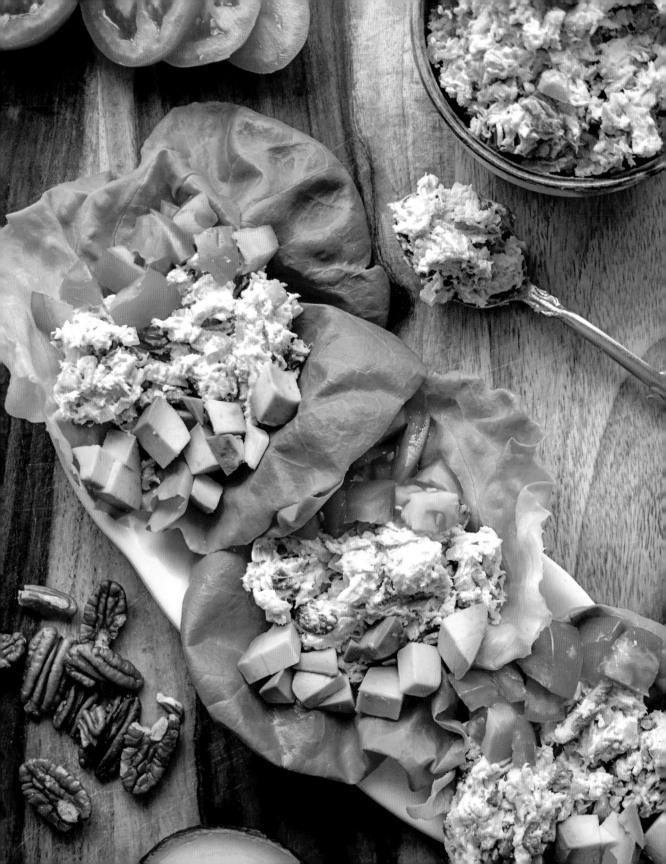

Chicken Salad Lettuce Wraps

Serves: 4 / Time: 15 minutes

INGREDIENTS

Chicken salad:

1 cooked rotisserie chicken

2 celery stalks, diced

½ cup avocado oil mayonnaise

¼ cup pecans, chopped

2 teaspoons apple cider vinegar

¼ teaspoon sea salt

¼ teaspoon freshly ground black pepper

Wrap assembly:

1 head butter lettuce

1 avocado, cubed

2 Roma tomatoes, diced

DIRECTIONS

Remove the bones from the chicken and chop or shred the meat.

In a large bowl, combine the chicken with the remaining salad ingredients and mix well.

Carefully remove several lettuce leaves, then rinse and dry them.

Fill each leaf with about ½ cup chicken salad. Top with the avocado and tomatoes. Roll up and serve.

MAKE IT VEGAN

Use shredded jackfruit instead of chicken.

GIVE IT A COLLAGEN BOOST

Stir 1 scoop of collagen protein into the chicken salad.

Nutrition information per serving: *675 calories, 58.2 g fat, 11.4 g saturated fat, 22.7 g protein, 10.4 g carbohydrate, 5.5 g fiber, 555 mg sodium*

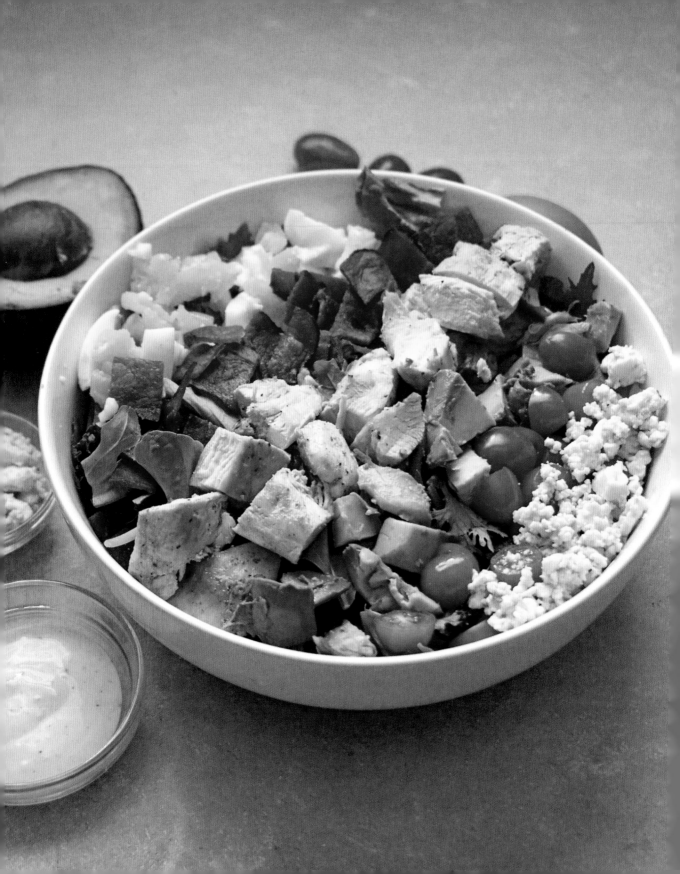

Cobb Salad

Serves: 2 / Time: 10 minutes

INGREDIENTS

4 cups spring greens

2 cooked boneless, skinless chicken breasts, cut into 1-inch pieces

4 pieces turkey or beef bacon, cooked and chopped

½ cup cherry tomatoes, sliced

¼ cup blue cheese crumbles

2 hard-boiled eggs, sliced

½ avocado, sliced

4 tablespoons Avocado Ranch Dressing (page 219)

DIRECTIONS

In a large bowl, combine all the ingredients, except the dressing, until well mixed. Divide between two bowls.

Top with 2 tablespoons of Avocado Ranch Dressing, or to taste, and serve.

MAKE IT DAIRY FREE

Omit the blue cheese crumbles.

Nutrition information per serving: *486 calories, 28.5 g fat, 6.4 g saturated fat, 47.9 g protein, 8.3 g carbohydrate, 6.2 g fiber, 602 mg sodium*

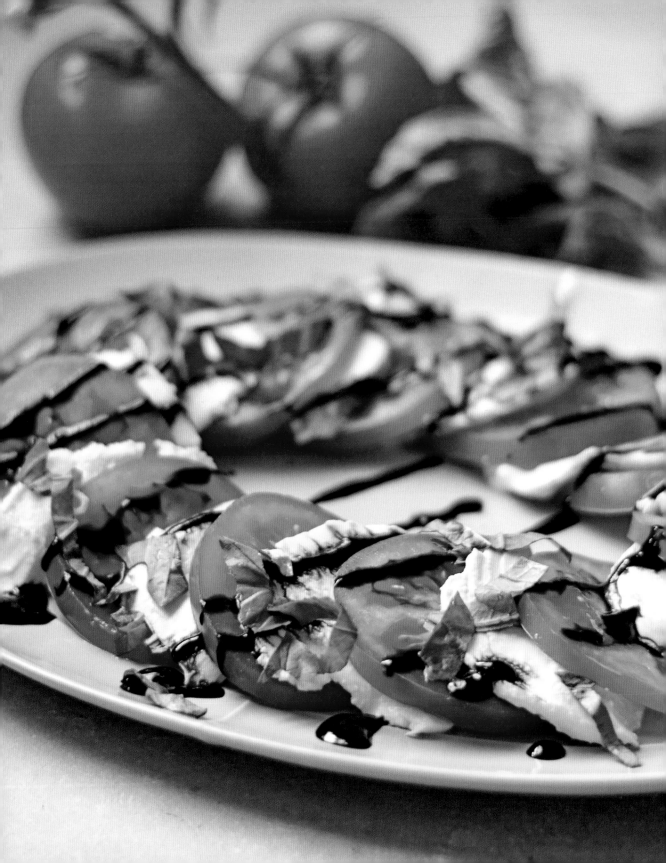

Caprese Salad

Serves: 8 / Time: 10 minutes

INGREDIENTS

8 ounces fresh
mozzarella cheese

4 tomatoes

¼ cup balsamic vinegar

¼ cup extra virgin olive oil

1 cup fresh basil

1 teaspoon sea salt

½ teaspoon freshly ground
black pepper

DIRECTIONS

Cut the mozzarella and tomatoes into ¼-inch-thick slices and arrange in an alternating pattern on a plate.

In a small bowl, mix the balsamic vinegar and olive oil. Drizzle on top of the mozzarella and tomatoes.

Stack the fresh basil and roll it into a tight log. Carefully cut into thin julienne slices, and toss over the salad.

Sprinkle the salt and pepper on top and enjoy.

Nutrition information per serving: *148 calories, 11.4 g fat, 3.9 g saturated fat, 8.6 g protein, 3.6 g carbohydrate, 0.8 g fiber, 408 mg sodium*

Egg Tahini Salad

Serves: 4 / Time: 5 minutes

INGREDIENTS

3 cups fresh greens

2 Roma tomatoes, diced

1 bell pepper, diced

½ cup sliced radishes

1 avocado, sliced

6 hard-boiled eggs

2 ounces Tahini Lemon Dressing (page 231)

DIRECTIONS

In a large bowl, combine the greens, tomatoes, bell pepper, radishes, and avocado.

Slice, chop, or quarter the eggs and place them on top of the salad.

Drizzle with the dressing and serve in individual bowls.

Nutrition information per serving: *355 calories, 28.3 g fat, 5.8 g saturated fat, 13.4 g protein, 16.8 g carbohydrate, 7.6 g fiber, 121 mg sodium*

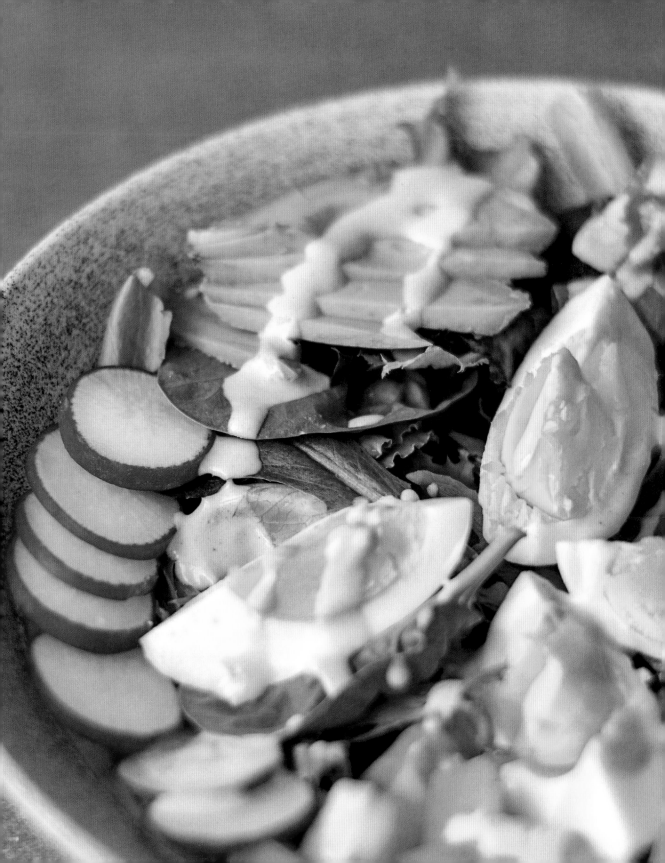

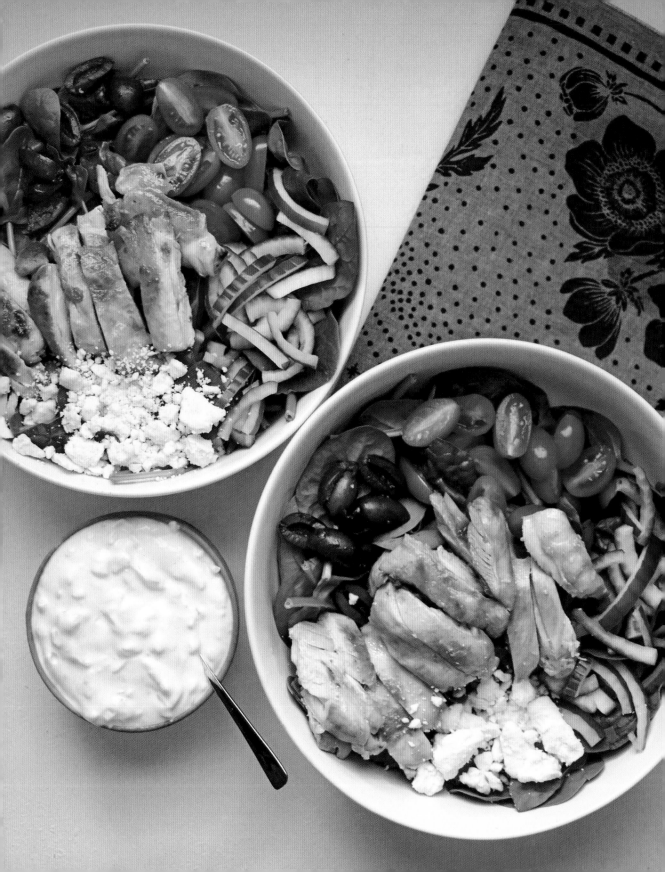

Mediterranean Chicken Salads with Tzatziki Sauce

Serves: 2 / Time: 1 hour

INGREDIENTS

Chicken:

3 tablespoons extra virgin olive oil, divided

Juice of ½ lemon

1 tablespoon organic apple cider vinegar

½ teaspoon garlic powder

1 pound (about 4) boneless, skinless chicken thighs

Tzatziki Sauce:

1 cup full-fat organic Greek yogurt

1 tablespoon extra virgin olive oil

½ cup deseeded and grated Persian cucumber

2 garlic cloves, minced

Juice of 1 lemon

¼ teaspoon sea salt

Salad:

3 to 4 cups baby spinach leaves

½ cup cherry tomatoes, sliced

½ red onion, sliced

¼ cup full-fat feta, crumbled

¼ cup Kalamata olives, sliced

DIRECTIONS

In a small bowl, mix together 2 tablespoons olive oil, lemon juice, cider vinegar, and garlic powder. Put the chicken thighs in a large bowl and pour the marinade over them. Put the chicken in the refrigerator to marinate for 30 minutes.

While the chicken marinates, mix together the tzatziki ingredients in a small bowl and set aside.

Heat the remaining 1 tablespoon olive oil in a large skillet over medium heat. Add the chicken, cooking the thighs on each side for 8 to 10 minutes, or until cooked through and the internal temperature reaches 165°F.

Remove the chicken from the skillet and slice each thigh into four or five pieces.

Combine the salad ingredients and serve in two bowls, topped with the chicken and tzatziki sauce.

Nutrition information per serving: *899 calories, 67.7 g fat, 18.7 g saturated fat, 61.1 g protein, 19.2 g carbohydrate, 3.2 g fiber, 1,375 mg sodium*

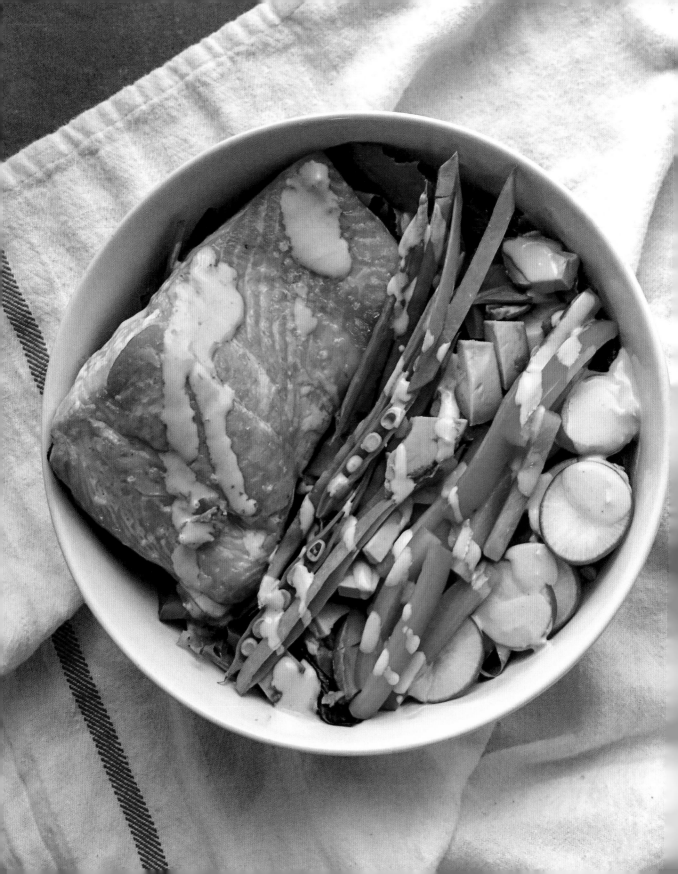

Salmon Salad

Serves: 1 / Time: 15 minutes

INGREDIENTS

1 teaspoon coconut oil

4 ounces wild-caught salmon fillet

¼ teaspoon sea salt

2 cups fresh greens

¼ cup sliced bell pepper

2 radishes, thinly sliced

¼ cup sliced sugar snap peas

½ avocado, diced

2 ounces Tahini Lemon Dressing (page 231), Cashew Caesar Dressing (page 220), or Avocado Ranch Dressing (page 219)

DIRECTIONS

Turn the broiler to high.

Heat the coconut oil in a medium ovenproof skillet over medium-high heat. Place the salmon skin-side down in the skillet.

Cook the salmon for 4 to 5 minutes, flip, sprinkle with the salt, and move to the broiler. Cook for 6 minutes and remove to a plate.

Meanwhile, in a large bowl, combine the greens, bell pepper, radishes, sugar snap peas, and avocado.

Serve the salad topped with the cooked salmon and drizzled with the desired dressing.

Nutrition information per serving: *891 calories, 57.3 g fat, 12.8 g saturated fat, 74.4 g protein, 28.2 g carbohydrate, 14.1 g fiber, 933 mg sodium*

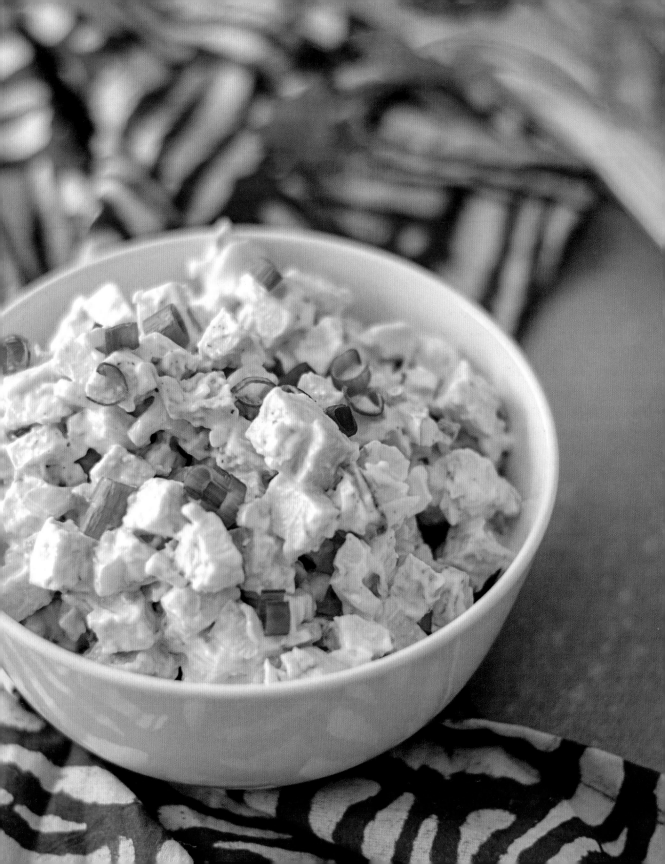

Turkey Salad

Serves: 4 / Time: 10 minutes

INGREDIENTS

1 pound turkey breast, cooked

3 green onions, sliced

2 celery stalks, diced

½ cup chopped walnuts

½ cup avocado oil mayonnaise

1 teaspoon fresh lemon juice

¼ teaspoon sea salt

¼ teaspoon freshly ground black pepper

Mixed greens

DIRECTIONS

Chop the turkey breast into small pieces.

In a large bowl, combine the turkey, onions, celery, walnuts, mayonnaise, lemon juice, salt, and pepper, and mix well.

Serve on a bed of mixed greens.

GIVE IT A COLLAGEN BOOST

Add 1 scoop of collagen protein.

Nutrition information per serving: *351 calories, 22.8 g fat, 2.2 g saturated fat, 31.8 g protein, 5.4 g carbohydrate, 2 g fiber, 254 mg sodium*

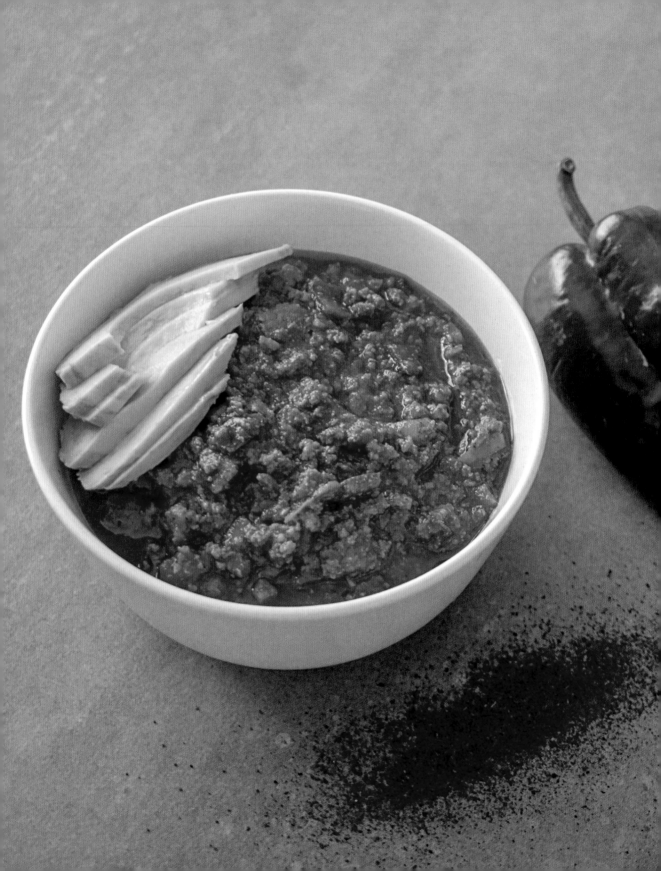

Buffalo Chili

Serves: 8 / Time: 1 hour, 20 minutes

INGREDIENTS

1 tablespoon coconut oil

2 pounds ground bison meat

1 large poblano pepper, diced

½ large onion, diced

3 garlic cloves, minced

1 (15-ounce) can roasted tomatoes

1 (15-ounce) can tomato sauce (no sugar added)

1 cup beef broth

¼ cup chili powder

1 tablespoon ground cumin

1 teaspoon sea salt

Toppings (optional):

Avocado

Grass-fed shredded cheese

Sour cream

DIRECTIONS

Heat the coconut oil in a large stockpot over medium heat. Add the bison meat and cook for 8 to 10 minutes, or until browned.

Add the pepper, onion, and garlic to the pot. Stir well and cook for 10 minutes. Stir in the tomatoes, tomato sauce, and broth. Add the chili powder, cumin, and salt.

Bring to a boil, stir well, reduce the heat to low, and cover. Let it simmer for about 1 hour, stirring occasionally.

Serve in bowls with the toppings (if using).

Nutrition information per serving: *192 calories, 10.8 g fat, 5 g saturated fat, 11.3 g protein, 14.2 g carbohydrate, 4.7 g fiber, 1,069 mg sodium*

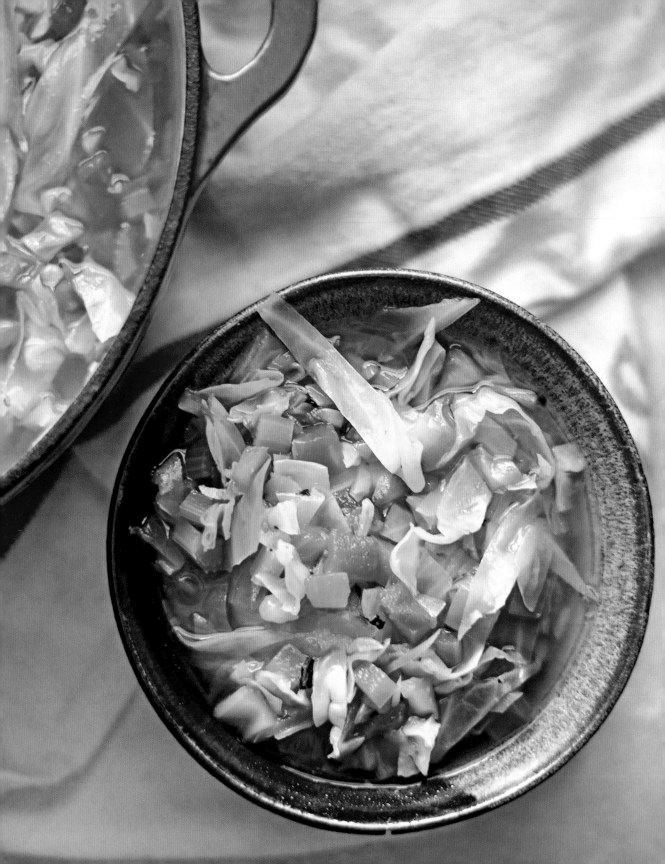

Cabbage Detox Soup

Serves: 8 / Time: 1 hour, 20 minutes

INGREDIENTS

1 tablespoon avocado oil

1 yellow onion, diced

1 cup diced celery

1 cup diced green bell pepper

4 garlic cloves, minced

1 tablespoon minced fresh turmeric

1 tablespoon minced fresh ginger

1 teaspoon freshly ground black pepper

1 tablespoon sea salt

1 small green cabbage, shredded

4 cups organic bone broth

4 cups filtered water

1 (14.5-ounce) can organic fire-roasted tomatoes

DIRECTIONS

Heat the avocado oil in a large pot over medium heat.

Add the onion, celery, bell pepper, garlic, turmeric, and ginger. Sauté for 5 to 7 minutes, or until the vegetables have softened. Stir in the black pepper and a pinch of the salt.

Add the cabbage and sauté 1 to 2 minutes. Stir in another pinch of salt.

Stir in the bone broth, water, tomatoes, and the remaining salt. Bring to a boil and cook for for 5 minutes. Reduce the heat to a low simmer, cover, and let simmer for about 1 hour, stirring about every 15 minutes. Serve warm.

MAKE IT VEGAN
Use vegetable stock instead of bone broth.

Nutrition information per serving: *63 calories, 0.3 g fat, 0.1 g saturated fat, 7.3 g protein, 8.3 g carbohydrate, 2.2 g fiber, 236 mg sodium*

Chicken Chorizo Chili

Serves: 8 / Time: 1 hour, 15 minutes

INGREDIENTS

1 tablespoon avocado oil

½ bell pepper, diced

½ yellow onion, diced

1 pound ground chicken

1 pound chicken chorizo sausage, chopped

1 (15-ounce) can organic fire-roasted tomatoes

6 ounces tomato paste

1½ cups bone broth or chicken stock

1 jalapeño, diced

¼ cup chili powder

3 tablespoons cumin

1 teaspoon cayenne

1 tablespoon sea salt

1 tablespoon apple cider vinegar

DIRECTIONS

Heat the avocado oil in a medium skillet over medium heat. Sauté the bell pepper and yellow onion for 4 to 5 minutes, or until the vegetables are tender.

Add the ground chicken and chicken sausage, and cook for 6 to 8 minutes, or until browned.

Add the fire-roasted tomatoes, tomato paste, and broth. Stir well.

Add the jalapeño, chili powder, cumin, cayenne, salt, and vinegar. Stir well and bring to a boil. Reduce the heat to low and simmer for 1 hour. Serve the chili in bowls.

Nutrition information per serving: *241 calories, 8.7 g fat, 2.1 g saturated fat, 27.3 g protein, 14.2 g carbohydrate, 4.7 g fiber, 1,680 mg sodium*

Creamy Cucumber Avocado Soup

Serves: 4 / Time: 5 minutes

INGREDIENTS

½ cucumber, peeled

1 ripe avocado

5 celery stalks

3 tablespoons lemon juice

¼ to ½ cup water

1 teaspoon sea salt

½ teaspoon freshly ground black pepper

2 ounces raw cheddar cheese or goat feta cheese, shredded

DIRECTIONS

Blend all the ingredients except the cheese together in a high-speed blender, using as much water as needed to achieve the desired consistency.

Serve chilled topped with the cheese.

Nutrition information per serving: *172 calories, 14.7 g fat, 5.2 g saturated fat, 5 g protein, 6.9 g carbohydrate, 4 g fiber, 580 mg sodium*

Chicken Vegetable Soup

Serves: 8 / Time: 45 minutes

INGREDIENTS

2 tablespoons avocado oil

2 garlic cloves, minced

½ large onion, diced

1 bell pepper, diced

2 celery stalks, diced

1 (32-ounce) carton chicken bone broth

4 cups water

2 tablespoons apple cider vinegar

1 pound boneless, skinless chicken breasts

1 (15-ounce) can tomatoes with green chilies

2 cups green beans, fresh or frozen

1 teaspoon sea salt

2 bay leaves

1 small bunch fresh thyme

2 cups shredded kale

DIRECTIONS

Heat the avocado oil in a large soup pot over medium heat. Sauté the garlic, onion, bell pepper, and celery for 5 minutes.

Add the bone broth, water, and vinegar. Stir well. Add the chicken, tomatoes, green beans, salt, bay leaves, and thyme.

Bring the soup to a boil, reduce the heat to low, and cover. Simmer for 25 minutes, or until the chicken has cooked through and the internal temperature reaches 165°F.

Carefully remove the chicken, shred it using two forks, and return it to the soup.

Remove the bay leaves and thyme, and stir in the kale. Add more sea salt to taste. When the kale has wilted a bit, the soup is ready to serve.

MAKE IT VEGAN

Omit the chicken and use vegetable broth in place of the chicken bone broth.

Nutrition information per serving: *162 calories, 2.7 g fat, 0.1 g saturated fat, 23.7 g protein, 10.3 g carbohydrate, 2 g fiber, 715 mg sodium*

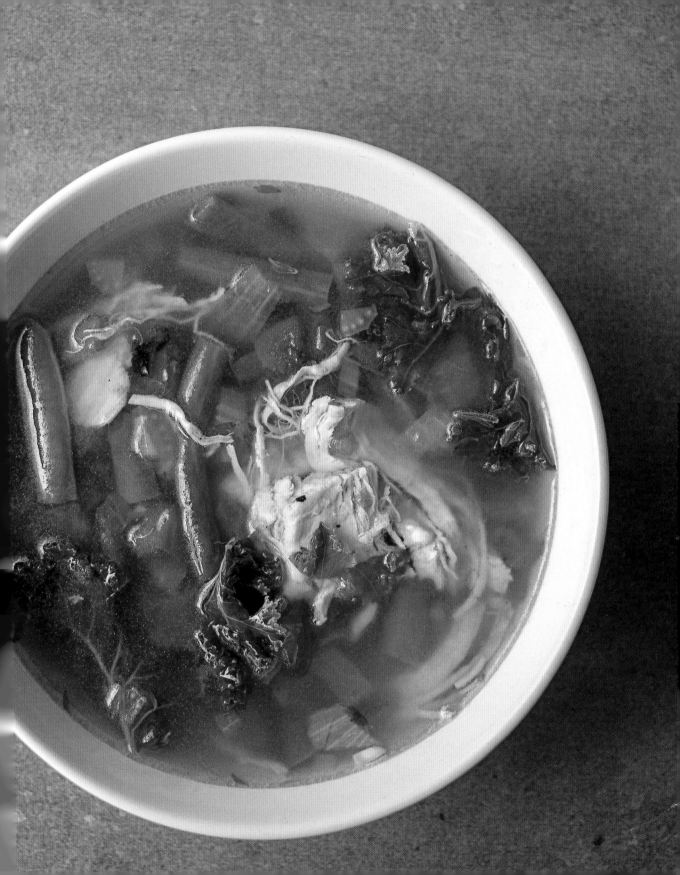

Lamb Stew

Serves: 6 / Time: 3 hours

INGREDIENTS

4 cups lamb or chicken broth

4 cups water

1 (32-ounce) can crushed tomatoes

1 bouquet garni package (thyme, oregano, parsley, bay leaf), tied with twine

1 large red onion, diced

1 tablespoon grapeseed oil

3 lamb shanks

1 lemon, halved and seeded

1 cup black olives, pitted

DIRECTIONS

In a large pot over medium-high heat, combine the broth, water, tomatoes, bouquet garni, and onion. Cover.

Heat the grapeseed oil in a large skillet over medium-high heat until shimmering. Add the lamb shanks and sear for 3 minutes on each side.

Add the seared lamb to the pot and bring almost to a boil. Reduce the heat to medium-low and simmer gently for 2 hours.

Squeeze the lemon juice directly into the pot. Add the lemon halves to the pot along with the olives. Cook uncovered for 15 minutes.

Remove from the heat and let the stew rest for 15 minutes.

Remove and discard the bouquet garni and lemon halves. Pull the meat from the bones. Discard the bones or save for making stock. Serve.

Nutrition information per serving: *327 calories, 14.6 g fat, 4.1 g saturated fat, 21.2 g protein, 26.8 g carbohydrate, 8.4 g fiber, 1613 mg sodium*

VARIATION:
Alternatively, sear the lamb and put it in a crockpot on low along with the broth, water, tomatoes, bouquet garni, onion, and oil. Cover and cook for 8 hours. Add the lemon juice and olives, cover, turn off the heat, remove the bouquet garni, and pull apart the meat before serving.

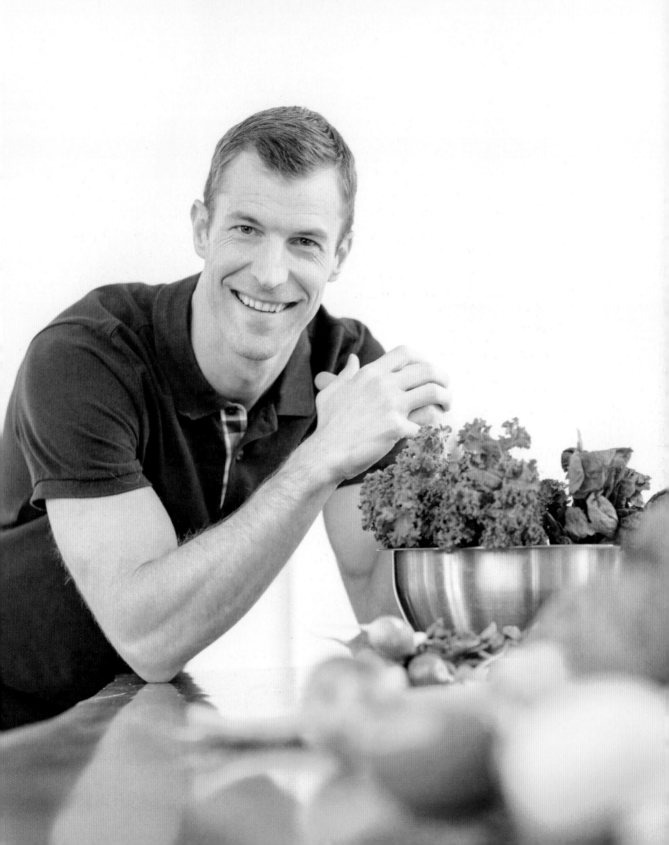

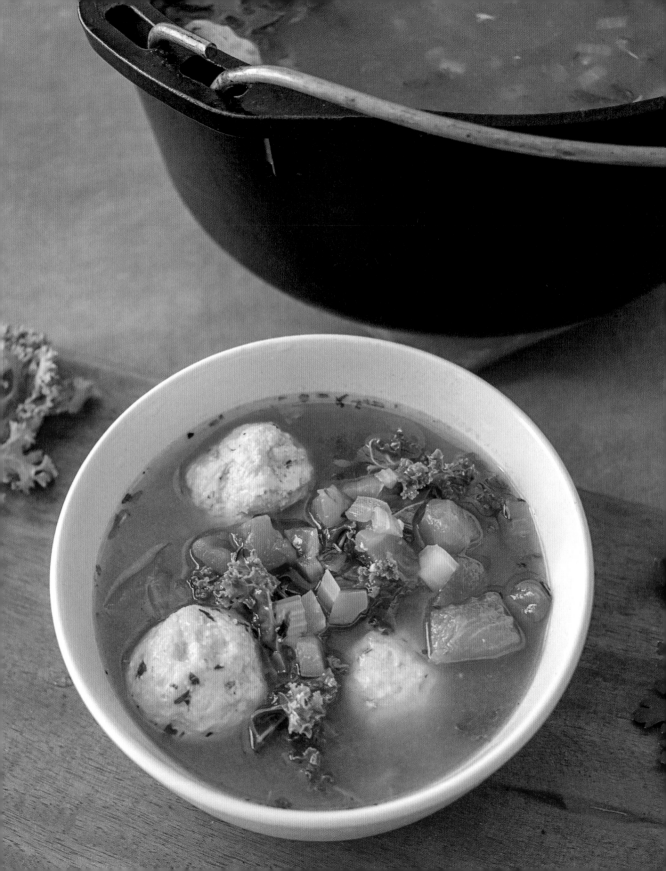

Turkey Meatball Soup

Serves: 8 / Time: 1 hour, 10 minutes

INGREDIENTS

Meatballs:

1 pound ground turkey

1 tablespoon coconut flour

½ cup finely chopped fresh parsley

2 large eggs

½ teaspoon sea salt

½ teaspoon garlic powder

Soup:

4 tablespoons avocado oil

4 celery stalks, diced

1 sweet onion, diced

1 bell pepper, diced

2 garlic cloves, minced

1 (32-ounce) carton chicken stock

2 cups water

1 (28-ounce) can diced tomatoes

1 tablespoon Italian seasoning

1 teaspoon sea salt

2 cups shredded fresh kale or spinach

¼ cup finely chopped fresh parsley

DIRECTIONS

Preheat the oven to 400°F. Line a baking sheet with parchment paper.

In a large bowl, combine all the meatball ingredients. Using clean hands, mix together well.

Scoop out tablespoonfuls of the meatball mixture, roll into balls, and place on the baking sheet, to make 40 small meatballs. Bake for 15 minutes, remove from the oven, and set aside.

Meanwhile, heat the avocado oil in a large soup pot over medium heat. Sauté the celery, onion, bell pepper, and garlic for 5 minutes, or until the vegetables are soft.

Pour in the chicken stock, water, tomatoes with their juice, Italian seasoning, and salt. Bring to a boil, reduce to a low simmer, and cover. Let the soup simmer for 30 to 45 minutes.

Remove the lid and add the cooked meatballs, kale, and parsley. Cook for 10 minutes, or until the meatballs are fully cooked through.

Nutrition information per serving: *261 calories, 12.6 g fat, 2.5 g saturated fat, 28.2 g protein, 13.2 g carbohydrate, 4.4 g fiber, 699 mg sodium*

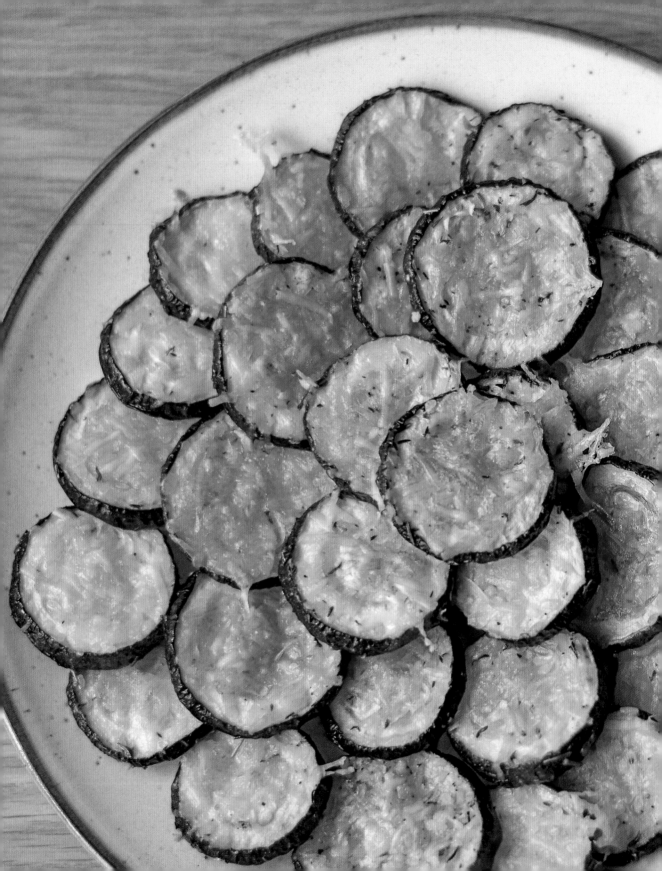

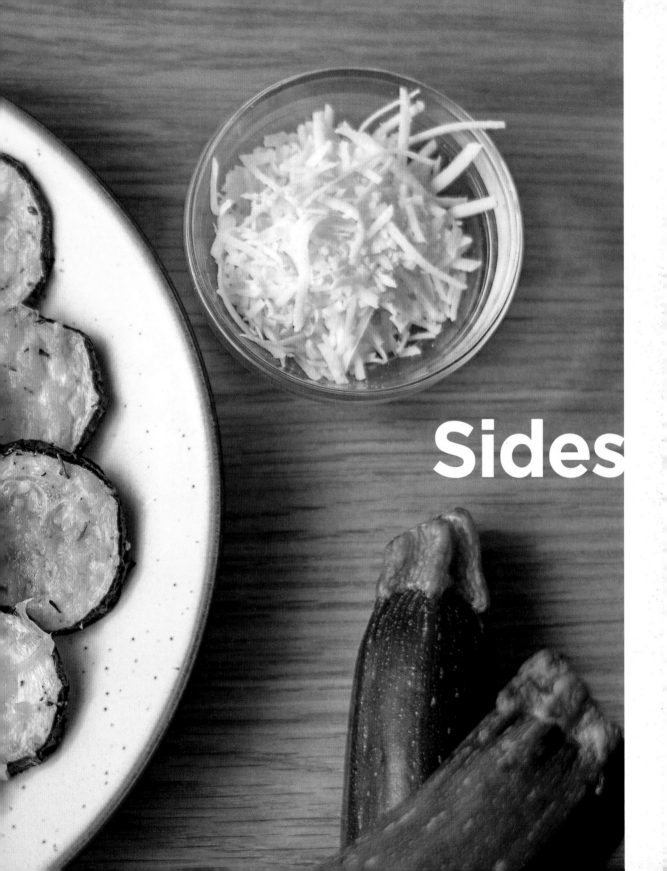

Sides

Asian-Inspired Green Beans

Serves: 2 / Time: 15 minutes

INGREDIENTS

2 teaspoons coconut oil

1 teaspoon toasted sesame oil

2 cups fresh green beans

2 tablespoons coconut aminos

DIRECTIONS

Heat the coconut oil and toasted sesame oil in a large skillet over medium heat. Add the green beans and sauté, tossing often, for 8 to 10 minutes, or until softened.

Add the coconut aminos and cook for 2 to 3 minutes, or until the aminos have slightly evaporated. Serve warm.

Nutrition information per serving: *108 calories, 6.9 g fat, 4.3 g saturated fat, 2 g protein, 10.8 g carbohydrate, 3.7 g fiber, 24 mg sodium*

Swiss Chard Greens

Serves: 6 / Time: 1 hour

INGREDIENTS

¼ **cup coconut oil**

2 **tablespoons minced garlic**

5 **cups chicken or vegetable stock**

5 **bunches Swiss chard, greens trimmed and chopped**

Sea salt and freshly ground black pepper, to taste

1 **tablespoon red pepper flakes**

DIRECTIONS

Melt the coconut oil in a large pot over medium-high heat.

Add the garlic and sauté for 2 to 3 minutes.

Pour in the chicken or vegetable stock, cover, and simmer for 30 minutes.

Add the greens to the pot and increase the heat to medium-high.

Cook the greens for 15 minutes, stirring occasionally.

Reduce the heat to medium and season with the salt and pepper. Cook until the greens are tender.

Drain the greens and add the red pepper flakes.

Serve immediately.

Nutrition information per serving: *267 calories, 12.9 g fat, 8.9 g saturated fat, 34.6 g protein, 2.6 g carbohydrate, 0.8 g fiber, 177 mg sodium*

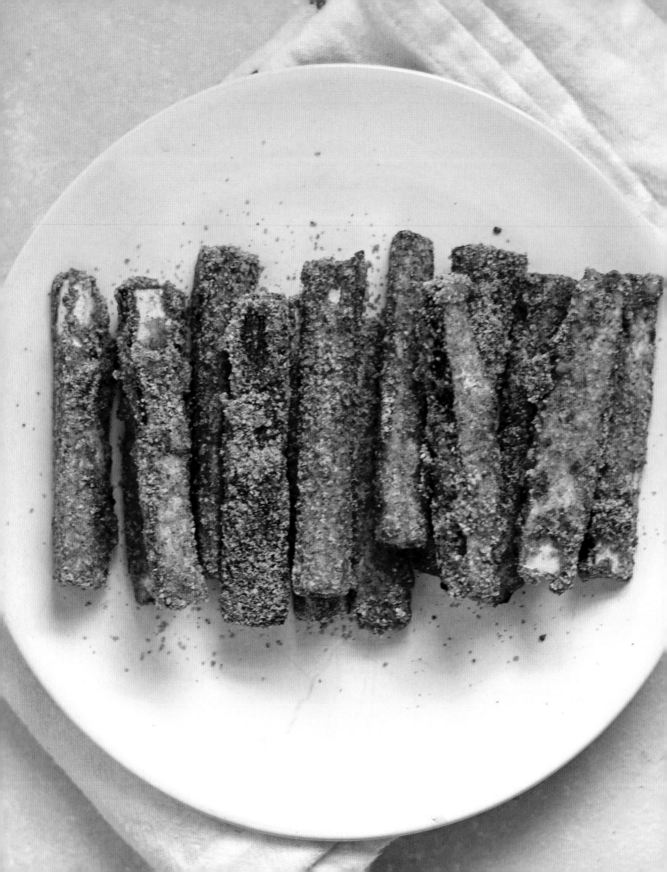

Baked Zucchini Fries

Serves: 2 / Time: 40 minutes

INGREDIENTS

1 large or 2 small zucchini

¼ cup almond flour

1 teaspoon paprika

½ teaspoon sea salt

1 large egg

DIRECTIONS

Preheat the oven to 375°F. Line a baking sheet with parchment paper.

Slice the zucchini into "fries." Set them on a paper towel to drain for 5 minutes.

In a small bowl, mix together the almond flour, paprika, and salt. In another bowl, whisk the egg.

Dip each zucchini piece first in the egg, then in the almond flour mixture. Place the fries on the prepared baking sheet.

Bake for 15 minutes. Carefully flip them and bake for 10 minutes, or until golden brown.

Serve warm.

Nutrition information per serving: *80 calories, 4.4 g fat, 0.9 g saturated fat, 5.6 g protein, 6.9 g carbohydrate, 2.6 g fiber, 174 mg sodium*

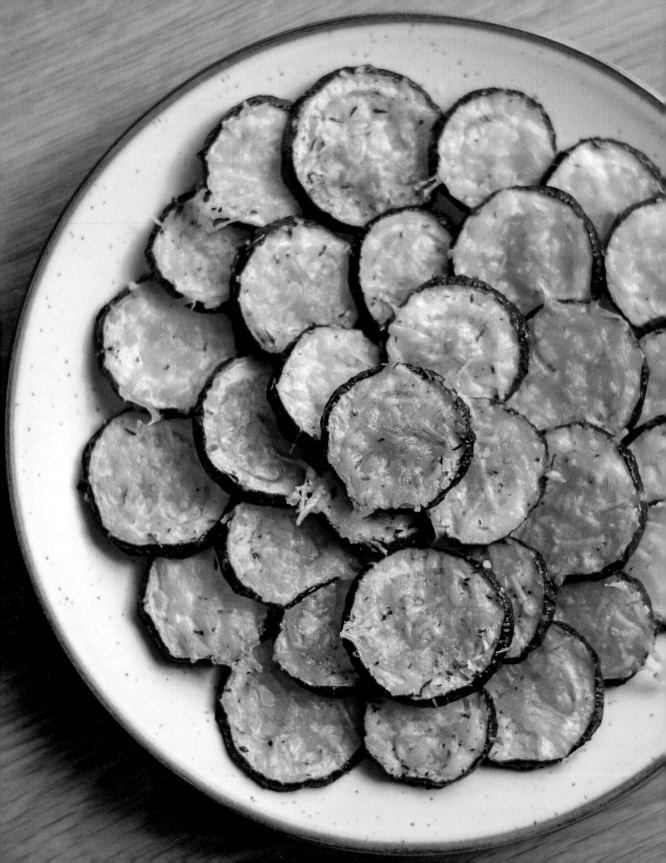

Baked Zucchini Slices

Serves: 4 / Time: 30 minutes

INGREDIENTS

2 zucchini

1 tablespoon avocado oil

1 teaspoon dried thyme

Sea salt and freshly ground black pepper, to taste

⅓ cup freshly grated Parmesan cheese (optional)

DIRECTIONS

Preheat the oven to 400°F.

Cut the zucchini crosswise into ¼-inch slices.

In a medium bowl, toss the zucchini with the avocado oil, thyme, sea salt, and pepper.

Arrange in a single layer on a baking sheet and top with the Parmesan (if using).

Bake for 20 minutes. If desired, finish under the broiler for about 1 minute to brown the cheese.

MAKE IT VEGAN AND DAIRY FREE
Use a dairy-free cheese on top instead of Parmesan, or simply omit.

Nutrition information per serving: *55 calories, 2.9 g fat, 1.6 g saturated fat, 4.6 g protein, 4 g carbohydrate, 1.3 g fiber, 205 mg sodium*

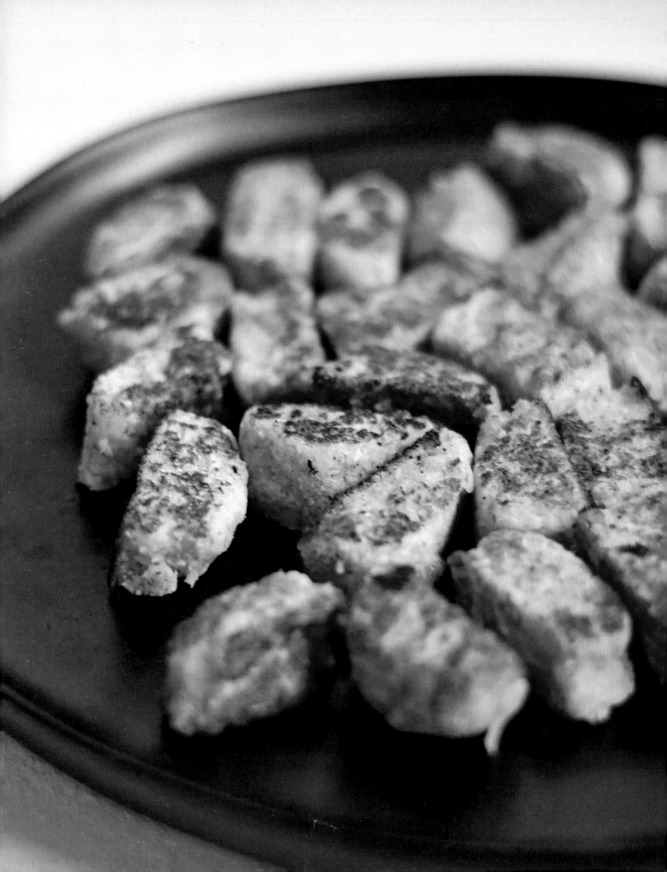

Cauliflower Gnocchi Bites

Serves: 4 / Time: 25 minutes

INGREDIENTS

2 cups riced cauliflower

¼ cup almond flour

¼ cup ground, whole
psyllium husk

1 large egg

1 tablespoon avocado oil

DIRECTIONS

In a small pot, heat the cauliflower rice for 5 to 6 minutes, until slightly warm.

Remove from the heat and stir in the almond flour and psyllium husk powder. Add the egg and mix well.

When the mixture resembles a dough, divide it into four pieces.

Carefully roll out each piece into a long, skinny log. Cut each log into eight ½-inch-thick pieces, making about 32 cauliflower gnocchi bites in all.

Heat a large skillet over medium-high heat and add the avocado oil. Cook the gnocchi for 3 to 4 minutes on each side, until crispy and cooked through. Don't crowd the skillet. Cook in batches if needed.

Nutrition information per serving: *78 calories, 2.4 g fat, 0.5 g saturated fat, 3.8 g protein, 10.7 g carbohydrate, 6.8 g fiber, 116 mg sodium*

Cheesy Broccoli

Serves: 4 / Time: 30 minutes

INGREDIENTS

1 pound broccoli florets (fresh or frozen)

4 tablespoons grass-fed butter, ghee, or coconut oil

½ teaspoon sea salt

1 cup shredded cheddar cheese

¼ cup freshly grated Parmesan cheese

DIRECTIONS

Preheat the oven to 400°F.

Bring 1 inch of water to a boil in a large pot over medium-high heat. Add in the broccoli, cover, and cook for 5 minutes.

Drain the broccoli and put it in a greased medium casserole dish.

Add the butter and mix it together well. Top with the salt and cheese.

Bake for 20 minutes, or until the cheese begins to brown.

MAKE IT VEGAN AND DAIRY FREE
Use coconut oil and dairy-free cheese.

Nutrition information per serving: *297 calories, 25.1 g fat, 18.9 g saturated fat, 12.9 g protein, 8.2 g carbohydrate, 3 g fiber, 525 mg sodium*

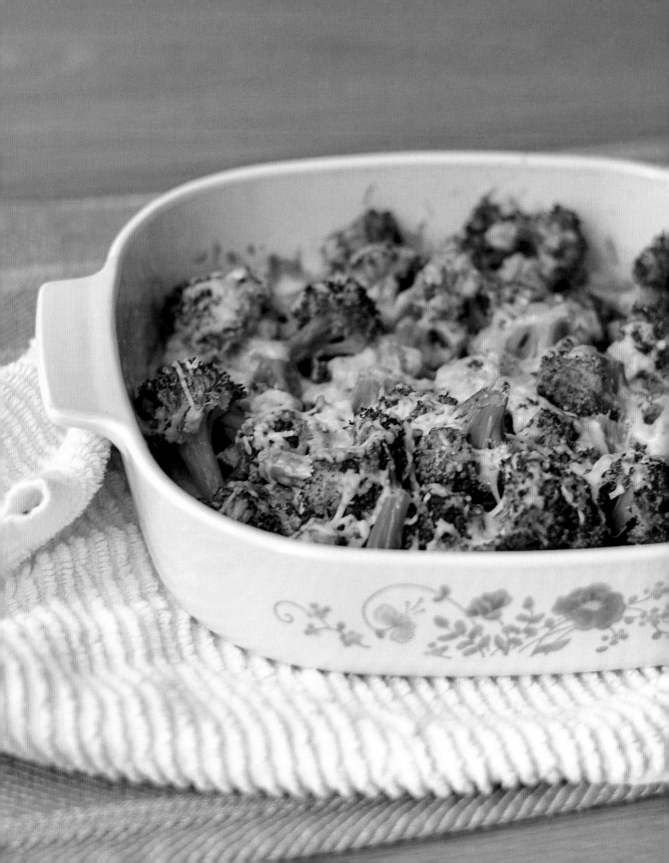

Chicken Liver Pâté

Serves: 8 / Time: 25 minutes

INGREDIENTS

3 tablespoons butter, plus 3 tablespoons, melted, for topping (optional)

3 garlic cloves

1 shallot, chopped

1 sprig rosemary

1 sprig thyme

1 teaspoon sea salt

1 teaspoon freshly ground black pepper

1 pound chicken livers

Gluten-free crostinis

DIRECTIONS

Heat 3 tablespoons of the butter in a saucepan over medium heat. Add the garlic, shallot, rosemary, thyme, salt, and pepper and sauté for 5 minutes.

Add the chicken livers and cook for 15 minutes, or until no longer pink.

Pour the chicken liver mixture into a food processor and blend until smooth.

Transfer the pâté to a serving dish and top with the 3 tablespoons melted butter (if using).

Put in the refrigerator for 1 to 2 hours to chill.

Serve on gluten-free crostinis.

Nutrition information per serving: *237 calories, 16.6 g fat, 8.9 g saturated fat, 18.9 g protein, 2.8 g carbohydrate, 0.6 g fiber, 453 mg sodium*

Parmesan
Roasted Cauliflower

Serves: 4 / Time: 35 minutes

INGREDIENTS

1 large cauliflower

1 tablespoon avocado oil

½ cup freshly grated
Parmesan cheese

1 teaspoon sea salt

DIRECTIONS

Preheat the oven to 425°F. Line a baking sheet with parchment paper.

Stem and chop the cauliflower. In a bowl, toss the cauliflower pieces in the avocado oil to coat evenly.

Put the cauliflower on the baking sheet. Sprinkle with the Parmesan and salt.

Place in the oven and roast for 25 to 30 minutes, or until golden brown.

Nutrition information per serving: *134 calories, 8 g fat, 5.1 g saturated fat, 12.6 g protein, 5 g carbohydrate, 1.8 g fiber, 472 mg sodium*

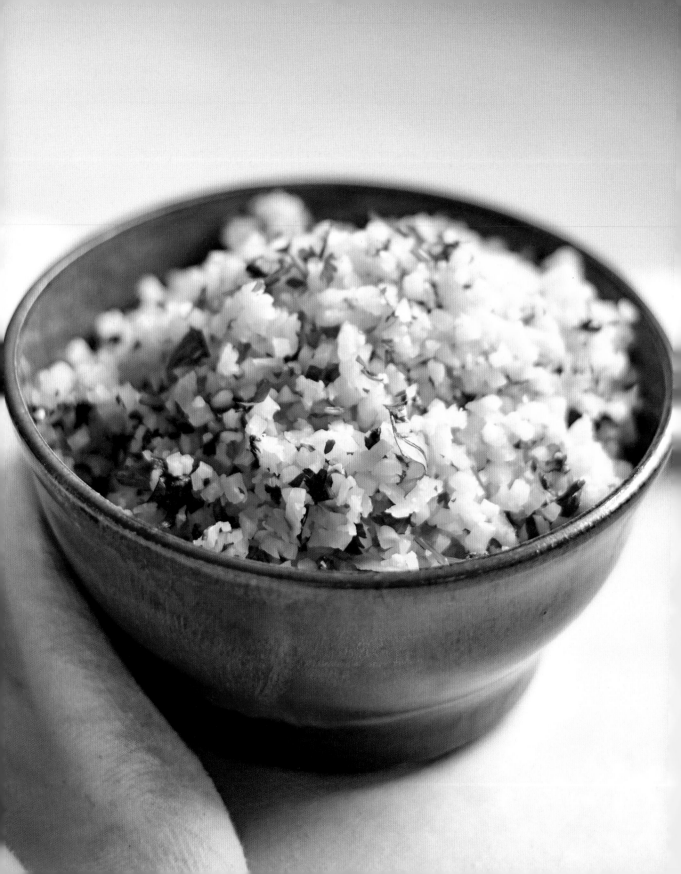

Cilantro Cauliflower Rice

Serves: 4 / Time: 15 minutes

INGREDIENTS

1 large cauliflower

1 tablespoon avocado oil

1 teaspoon sea salt

1 bunch cilantro, chopped

DIRECTIONS

Remove the stem and chop the cauliflower. Put it in a food processor and pulse several times, until the cauliflower has an almost rice-like texture.

Heat a large skillet over medium heat and add the avocado oil. Add the riced cauliflower and cook for about 10 minutes, until softened.

Stir in the salt and cilantro.

Remove from the heat and serve warm.

Nutrition information per serving: *58 calories, 0.7 g fat, 0.1 g saturated fat, 4.3 g protein, 11.5 g carbohydrate, 5.5 g fiber, 192 mg sodium*

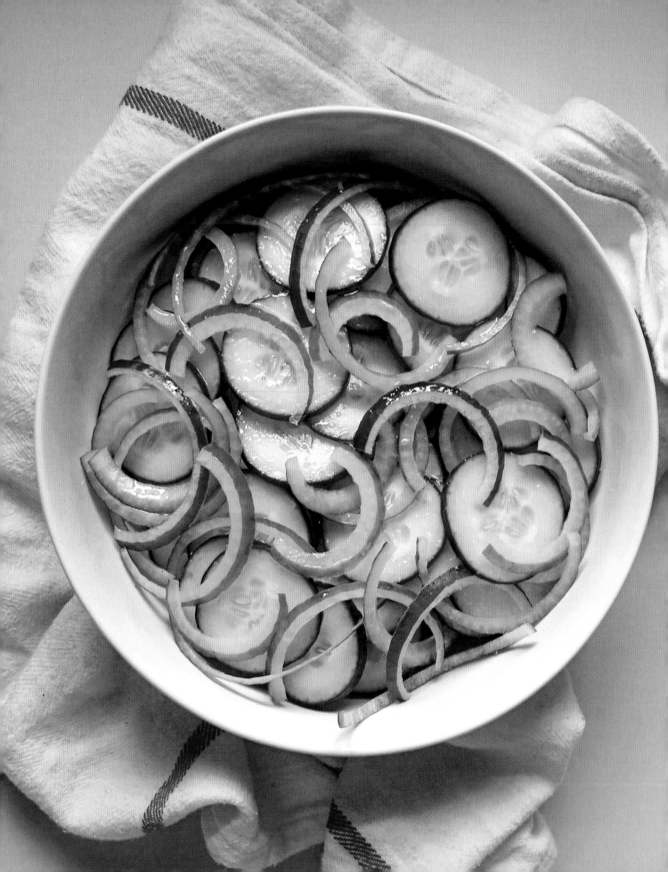

Cold Cucumber Salad

Serves: 2 / Time: 35 minutes

INGREDIENTS

1 large hothouse or English cucumber

¼ red onion, finely sliced

2 tablespoons organic apple cider vinegar

2 tablespoons extra virgin olive oil

5 drops liquid stevia

1 teaspoon sea salt

DIRECTIONS

Slice the cucumber and place in a medium bowl. Add the red onion.

In a small bowl, mix the apple cider vinegar, olive oil, stevia, and salt together. Pour over the cucumbers and onion.

Stir together well to combine and refrigerate for 30 minutes. Serve chilled.

Nutrition information per serving: *151 calories, 14.2 g fat, 2.1 g saturated fat, 1.1 g protein, 6.9 g carbohydrate, 1 g fiber, 254 mg sodium*

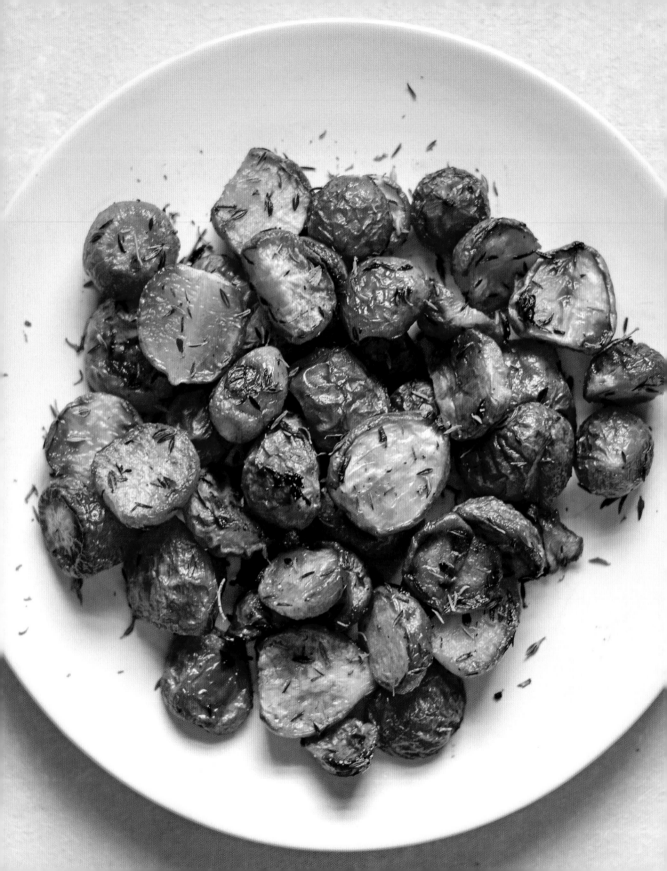

Roasted Radishes

Serves: 4 / Time: 45 minutes

INGREDIENTS

2 bunches red radishes

1 tablespoon avocado oil

2 teaspoons dried thyme

1 teaspoon sea salt

DIRECTIONS

Preheat the oven to 425°F.

Stem and clean the radishes.

Slice them in half and toss in the avocado oil, thyme, and salt. Place on a baking sheet.

Roast in the oven for 40 minutes, stirring them halfway through.

Serve warm.

Nutrition information per serving: *15 calories, 0.5 g fat, 0.1 g saturated fat, 0.5 g protein, 2.5 g carbohydrate, 1.3 g fiber, 150 mg sodium*

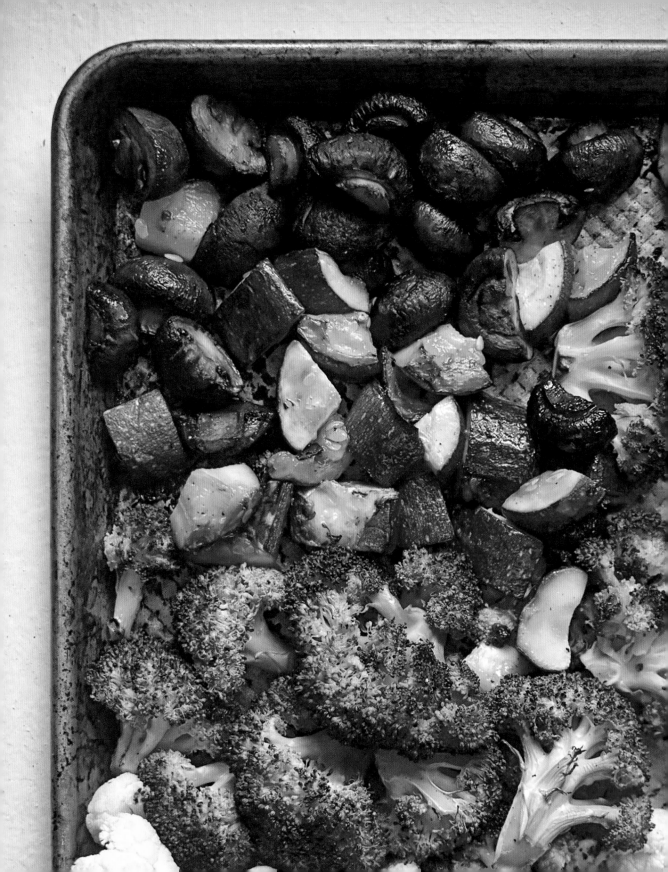

Roasted Vegetable Tray

Serves: 4 / Time: 45 minutes

INGREDIENTS

9 ounces broccoli

1 medium cauliflower

1 small zucchini

1 cup crimini mushrooms

2 tablespoons avocado oil

1 teaspoon sea salt

½ teaspoon freshly ground black pepper

DIRECTIONS

Preheat the oven to 425°F.

Stem and chop the broccoli and cauliflower into florets.

Chop the zucchini and the mushrooms into evenly sized pieces.

Put the vegetables in a large bowl and toss with the avocado oil, salt, and pepper. Transfer the vegetables to a rimmed baking sheet.

Place in the oven and roast for 15 minutes.

Stir the vegetables and bake for 15 to 20 minutes, or until they are roasted to your liking. Serve warm.

Nutrition information per serving: *55 calories, 1 g fat, 0.2 g saturated fat, 4.5 g protein, 9.6 g carbohydrate, 4.7 g fiber, 170 mg sodium*

Sautéed Spinach

Serves: 4 / Time: 12 minutes

INGREDIENTS

1 tablespoon avocado oil

1 garlic clove, minced

12 ounces fresh baby spinach (see Note)

Juice of ½ lemon

Sea salt, to taste

DIRECTIONS

Put the oil and garlic in a large skillet over medium heat.

Sauté the garlic for 1 to 2 minutes, until fragrant and slightly browned.

Add the spinach (it will fill the skillet completely but will cook down) and toss gently in the oil and garlic mixture. Cover for 5 minutes to wilt the spinach.

Remove the lid and stir well.

Remove from the heat, toss with the lemon juice, and add the salt. Serve immediately.

NOTE: This recipe also works with 1 pound of frozen spinach. Follow the directions on the package for stovetop cooking, and drain all excess liquid. Use as you would fresh spinach.

Nutrition information per serving: *27 calories, 0.5 g fat, 0.1 g saturated fat, 2.2 g protein, 4 g carbohydrate, 2.2 g fiber, 124 mg sodium*

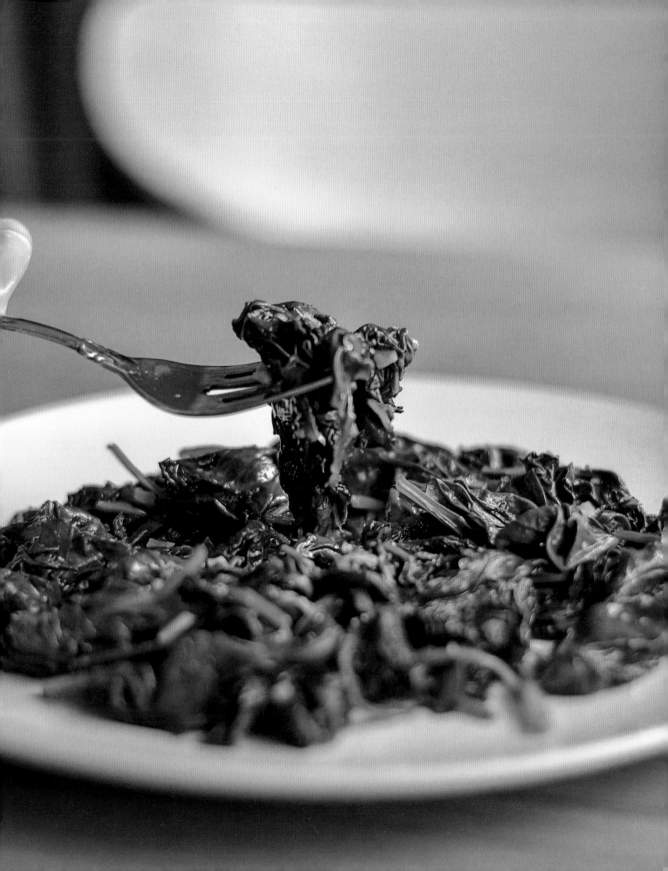

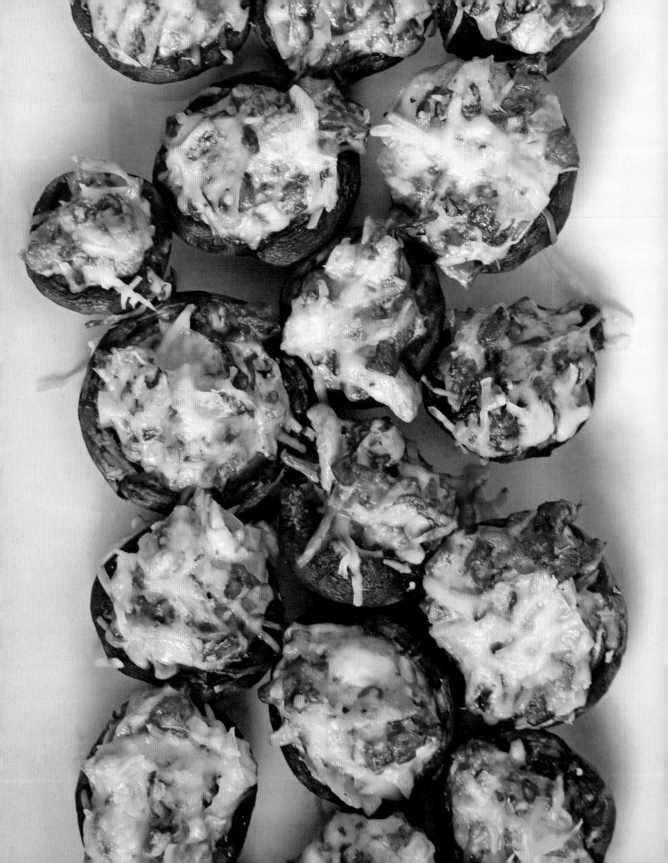

Stuffed Mushrooms

Serves: 6 / Time: 40 minutes

INGREDIENTS

2 cups whole baby bella mushrooms

1 tablespoon avocado oil

1 cup chopped fresh spinach

½ cup chopped artichoke hearts

2 garlic cloves, minced

2 tablespoons unsweetened almond milk

3 tablespoons avocado oil mayonnaise

1 teaspoon chopped fresh parsley

½ teaspoon sea salt

Freshly grated Parmesan cheese (optional)

DIRECTIONS

Preheat the oven to 350°F. Line a baking sheet with parchment paper.

Carefully remove the stems from the mushrooms. Set aside the mushroom caps and finely dice the stems.

Heat the avocado oil in a skillet over medium heat. Add the mushroom stems, spinach, artichoke hearts, and garlic. Sauté for 5 minutes, or until the spinach has wilted and the mushroom stems are softened.

Add the almond milk and cook for 1 minute.

Remove from the heat and stir in the mayonnaise, parsley, and salt.

Scoop the mixture into the mushroom caps and place on the baking sheet. Sprinkle on the cheese, if using. Bake the mushrooms for 20 to 22 minutes, or until they have softened.

MAKE IT VEGAN
Use a vegan mayonnaise.

MAKE IT DAIRY FREE
Omit the Parmesan cheese.

Nutrition information per serving: *158 calories, 7.1 g fat, 1.5 g saturated fat, 10 g protein, 18.4 g carbohydrate, 8.5 g fiber, 257 mg sodium*

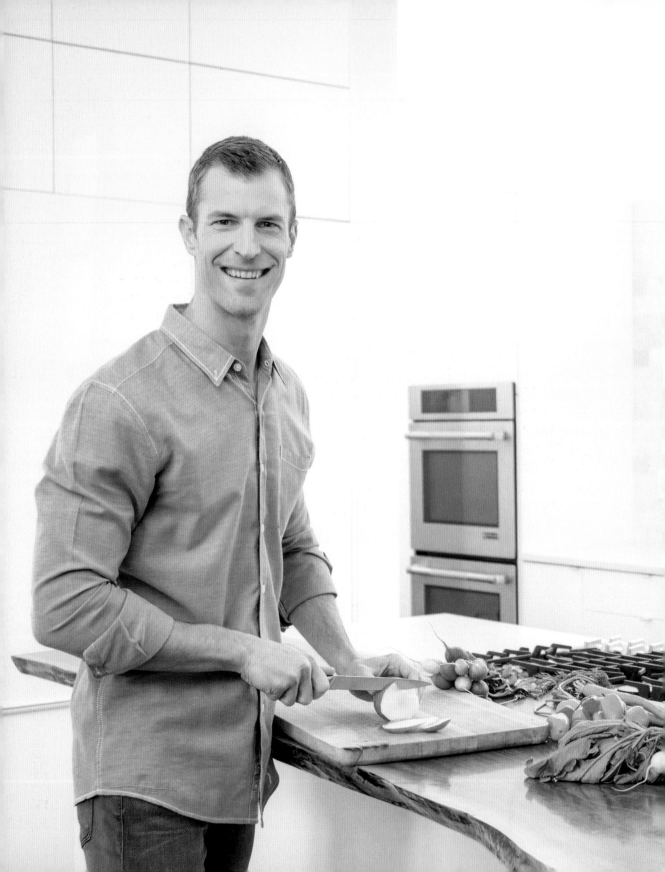

Twice-Baked Cauliflower

Serves: 6 / Time: 40 minutes

INGREDIENTS

1 large cauliflower

2 ounces organic cream cheese, softened

¼ cup full-fat organic Greek yogurt

¼ cup freshly grated Parmesan cheese

½ teaspoon sea salt

¼ cup cheddar cheese, for topping (optional)

Cooked beef or turkey bacon, for topping (optional)

DIRECTIONS

Stem and chop the cauliflower. Put 1 to 2 inches of water in a large pot and bring to a boil. Add the cauliflower, cover, and reduce the heat to a simmer. Let cook for 10 minutes, or until the cauliflower is soft. Drain the cauliflower and place in a large mixing bowl.

Preheat the oven to 375°F.

Mash the cauliflower with a fork or potato masher. Add the cream cheese, Greek yogurt, Parmesan, and salt. Mix well.

Put the mixture in a small ovenproof baking dish and top with the cheddar, if using. Bake for 20 minutes.

Top with the cooked beef or turkey bacon, if using, and serve.

Nutrition information per serving: *110 calories, 7 g fat, 3.9 g saturated fat, 8.4 g protein, 3.3 g carbohydrate, 1.1 g fiber, 289 mg sodium*

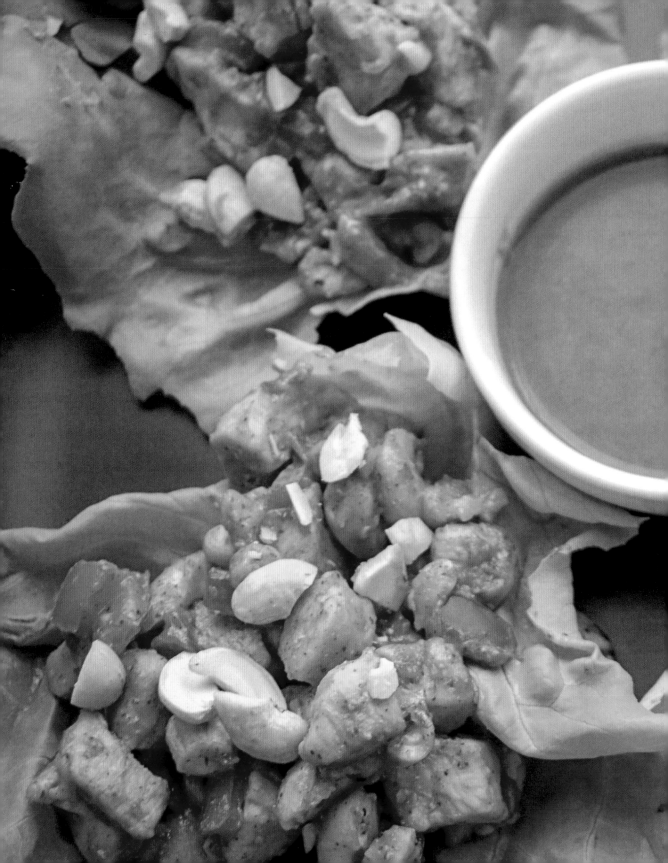

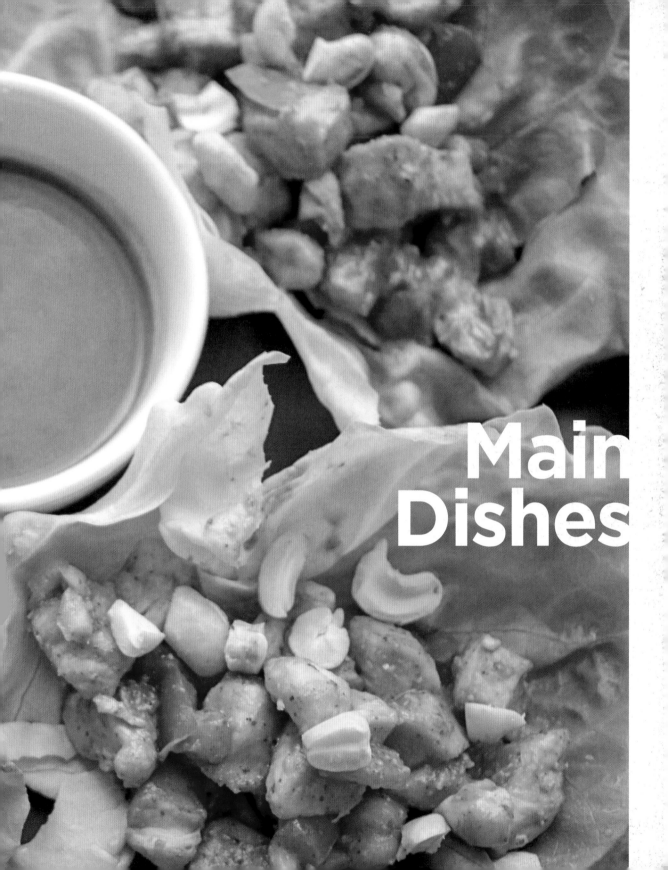

Main
Dishes

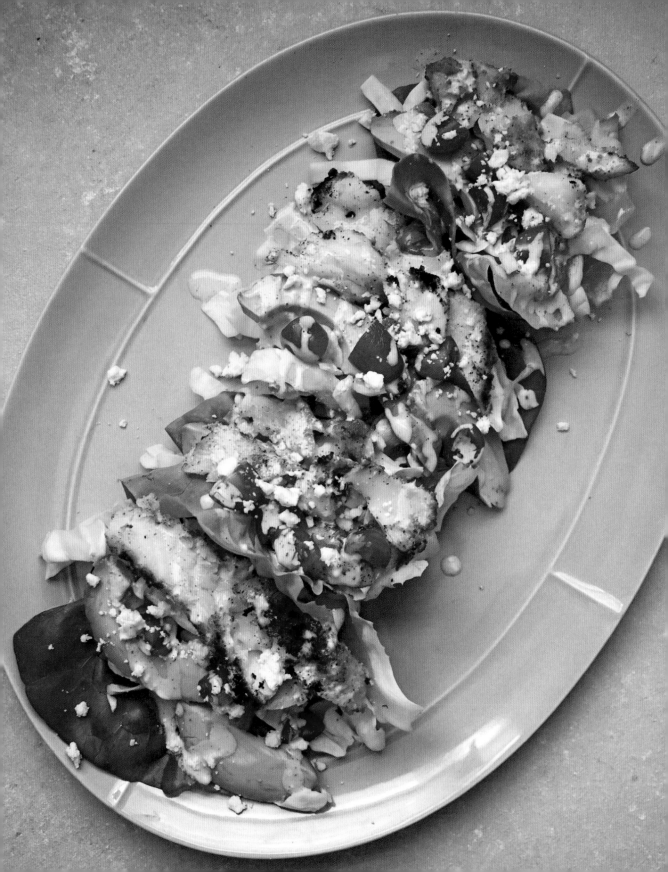

Baja Fish "Tacos"

Serves: 2 / Time: 30 minutes

INGREDIENTS

Fish:

3 tablespoons coconut flour

½ teaspoon chili powder

½ teaspoon sea salt

2 wild-caught cod fillets

1 tablespoon avocado oil

Baja Sauce:

¼ cup avocado oil mayonnaise

1 tablespoon fresh lime juice

1 tablespoon hot sauce

½ teaspoon chili powder

½ teaspoon sea salt

Toppings:

Bibb lettuce leaves, for taco cups

Queso fresco, crumbled

1 avocado, sliced

Cherry tomatoes, halved

Cabbage, shredded

DIRECTIONS

In a small bowl, mix the coconut flour together with the chili powder and salt. Dredge the fish pieces in it to cover.

Heat a skillet over medium-high heat and add the avocado oil. Pan-fry the fish for 4 to 5 minutes on each side, or until cooked through. Place the fish on a plate and cut into long strips.

In a small bowl, whisk together the mayonnaise, lime juice, hot sauce, chili powder, and sea salt for the Baja sauce.

Fill the lettuce cups with the fish strips and top with the sauce and toppings, as desired.

Nutrition information per serving: *576 calories, 41.4 g fat, 8.6 g saturated fat, 26.6 g protein, 28.1 g carbohydrate, 17.4 g fiber, 641 mg sodium*

Cheesy Poblano Casserole

Serves: 6 / Time: 1 hour

INGREDIENTS

3 poblano peppers

6 ounces goat feta cheese, crumbled

8 ounces beef bacon, chopped and cooked

3 cups cauliflower, riced

¼ cup green onions, chopped

½ cup chicken bone broth

1 cup mushrooms, diced

1 cup tomato sauce

1 teaspoon garlic powder

1 teaspoon onion powder

1 teaspoon cumin

2 tablespoons fresh dill, chopped

1 teaspoon sea salt

1 teaspoon freshly ground black pepper

1 cup grated Pecorino Romano, for topping

Avocado slices, for topping

Fresh cilantro, chopped, for topping

DIRECTIONS

Remove and discard the pepper stems. Slice the peppers in half lengthwise and remove the seeds and white veins inside.

Place the peppers cut-side down on a baking sheet and broil for about 10 minutes, flipping halfway through. Set aside.

Preheat the oven to 350°F.

Chop the peppers and place them in a large bowl.

Add the remaining ingredients, except for the toppings. Mix until well combined.

Pour the mixture into a casserole dish and top with the grated Pecorino.

Bake for 40 minutes.

Top with the avocado and cilantro and serve.

Nutrition information per serving: *499 calories, 28.2 g fat, 15.7 g saturated fat, 31.4 g protein, 13 g carbohydrate, 6.2 g fiber, 1,877 mg sodium*

Baked Italian Chicken

Serves: 4 / Time: 45 to 60 minutes

INGREDIENTS

2 tablespoons coconut oil

1 onion, chopped

1 cup mushrooms, sliced

8 ounces goat cheese (chèvre)

½ cup chicken stock

1 tomato, chopped

1 (14-ounce) can artichoke hearts, a few reserved for garnish (optional)

1 cup fresh spinach

½ teaspoon garlic powder

½ teaspoon Italian seasoning

Sea salt and freshly ground black pepper, to taste

4 bone-in, skin-on chicken breasts

DIRECTIONS

Preheat the oven to 350°F.

Heat the coconut oil in a large skillet over medium-high heat. Add the the onion and mushrooms and cook until tender.

Remove the veggies from the skillet to a bowl. Set aside.

Return the skillet to medium heat and add the goat cheese and the chicken stock. Stir until well combined.

Return the onion and mushrooms to the skillet and add the tomato, artichokes, spinach, garlic powder, Italian seasoning, and salt and pepper. Stir to combine. Cook until the spinach is slightly wilted.

Place the chicken breasts in a greased baking dish. Pour the veggie mixture over the chicken.

Bake the chicken for 30 minutes, or until the internal temperature reaches 165°F. Serve immediately.

Nutrition information per serving: *485 calories, 28.1 g fat, 14.1 g saturated fat, 49.8 g protein, 7.5 g carbohydrate, 1.7 g fiber, 662 mg sodium*

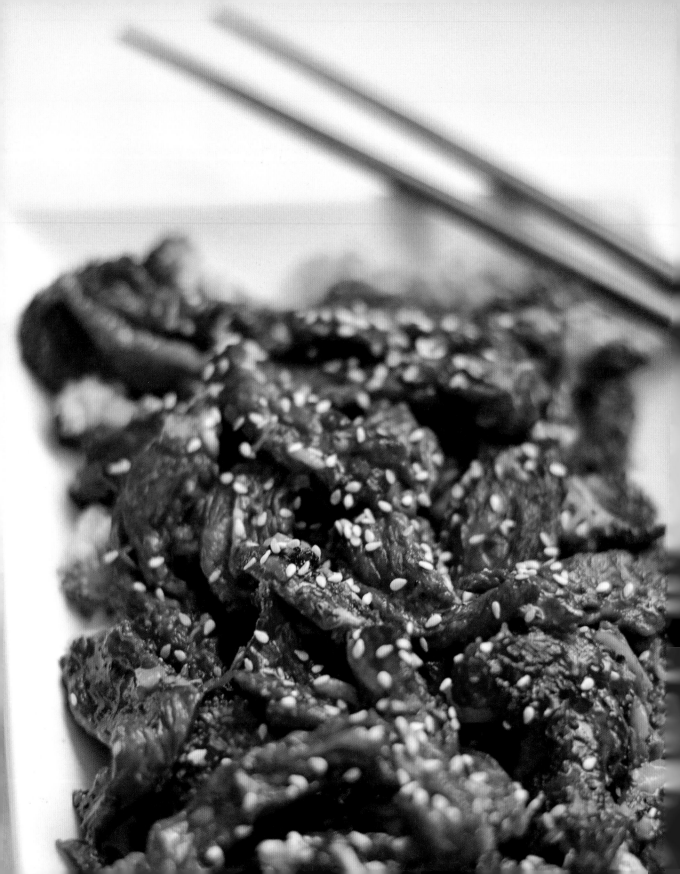

Beef and Broccoli

Serves: 4 / Time: 30 minutes

INGREDIENTS

1 pound beef flank or skirt steak

1 tablespoon coconut oil

½ inch fresh ginger, peeled and minced

4 cups broccoli florets

Sauce:

¼ cup coconut aminos

1 tablespoon arrowroot powder

2 teaspoons Thai fish sauce

1 teaspoon toasted sesame oil

5 to 10 drops liquid stevia (optional)

DIRECTIONS

Slice the flank steak into thin slices.

Heat the coconut oil in a large pan over medium-high heat. Add the ginger and stir quickly.

Add the beef and cook for 8 to 10 minutes, or until the beef is cooked through.

In a large pot, bring 2 to 3 inches of water to a boil. Steam the broccoli until fork-tender.

In a small bowl, stir together the sauce ingredients.

Add half of the broccoli to the pan with the meat and pour the sauce over it. Reduce the heat to low and stir until the sauce has thickened.

Put the remaining broccoli on plates and serve the flank steak and broccoli mixture over it.

Nutrition information per serving: *330 calories, 16.2 g fat, 7.5 g saturated fat, 33.2 g protein, 11.4 g carbohydrate, 2.4 g fiber, 457 mg sodium*

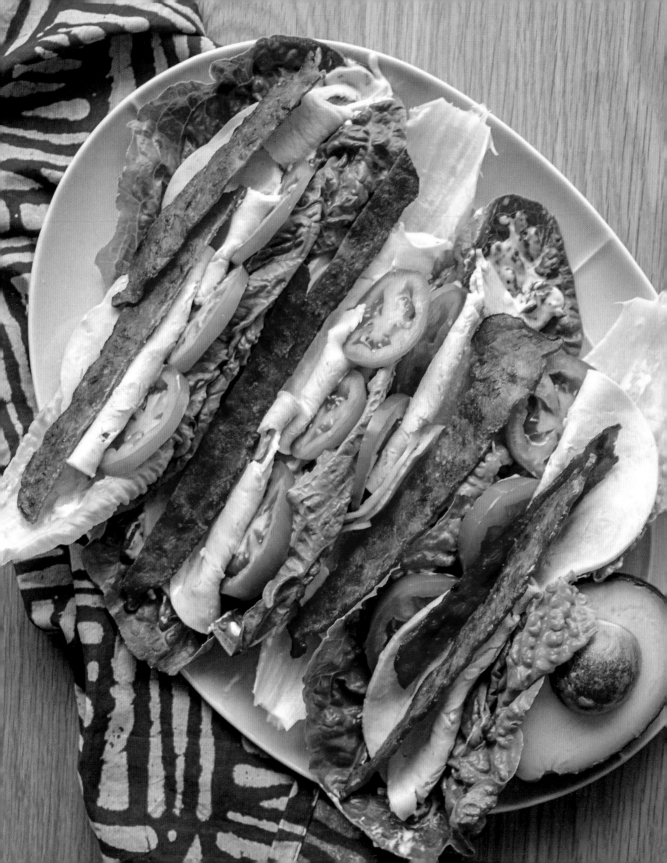

BLT Turkey Wrap

Serves: 4 / Time: 10 minutes

INGREDIENTS

½ **cup avocado oil mayonnaise**

1 teaspoon dried basil

½ teaspoon sea salt

¼ teaspoon freshly ground black pepper

8 romaine lettuce leaves

1 pound sliced turkey breast

8 slices turkey bacon, cooked

2 Roma tomatoes, sliced

DIRECTIONS

In a small bowl, combine the mayonnaise, basil, salt, and pepper.

Spread an equal amount of the mayonnaise mixture inside each romaine leaf.

Fill each romaine leaf with an equal amount of the turkey breast, bacon, and tomatoes.

Serve and enjoy.

Nutrition information per serving: *271 calories, 14 g fat, 1.9 g saturated fat, 26 g protein, 7.6 g carbohydrate, 1.4 g fiber, 1,714 mg sodium*

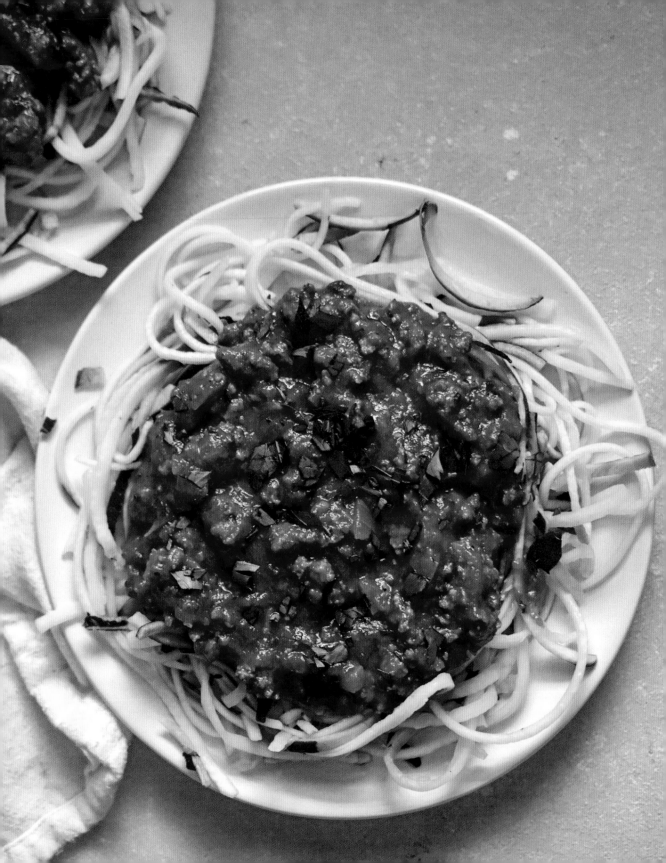

Bolognese and Zoodles

Serves: 4 / Time: 50 minutes

INGREDIENTS

1 tablespoon extra virgin olive oil

½ yellow onion, diced

2 celery stalks, diced

2 garlic cloves, minced

1 pound ground beef

1 (24-ounce) can crushed tomatoes, strained

3 tablespoons fresh parsley, finely chopped

2 teaspoons salt

1 teaspoon dried basil

2 large zucchini, spiralized into "zoodles"

DIRECTIONS

Heat a large skillet over medium heat and add the olive oil. Sauté the onion, celery, and garlic for 4 to 5 minutes, or until the onions are translucent.

Add the ground beef and cook for 8 to 10 minutes, until browned and cooked through.

Stir in the crushed tomatoes, parsley, salt, and basil. Reduce the heat to low and simmer for 30 minutes, stirring regularly.

Serve over the raw zucchini zoodles.

Nutrition information per serving: *345 calories, 10.9 g fat, 3.2 g saturated fat, 40.8 g protein, 21.2 g carbohydrate, 7.8 g fiber, 1589 mg sodium*

Tomato
Balsamic Chicken

Serves: 4 / Time: 50 minutes

INGREDIENTS

4 Roma tomatoes, diced

¼ red onion, finely diced

½ cup chopped fresh basil

2 tablespoons balsamic vinegar

2 garlic cloves, minced

1 tablespoon avocado oil

1½ pounds boneless, skinless chicken breasts

1 teaspoon sea salt

½ cup shredded organic mozzarella cheese (optional)

DIRECTIONS

Preheat the oven to 375°F.

In a large bowl, combine the tomatoes, onion, basil, vinegar, and garlic. Set aside.

Heat a large skillet over medium-high heat and add the avocado oil. Carefully add the chicken breasts and cook for 2 minutes on each side.

Remove the chicken from the skillet to an ovenproof casserole dish.

Sprinkle the chicken with the salt and mozzarella, if using. Spread half of the tomato mixture over the chicken. Bake the chicken for 30 minutes, or until the internal temperature reaches 165°F.

Remove from the oven and top with the remaining tomato mixture. Serve warm.

MAKE IT DAIRY FREE
Omit the cheese or use a dairy-free mozzarella cheese.

Nutrition information per serving: *367 calories, 14 g fat, 4 g saturated fat, 51.6 g protein, 6.4 g carbohydrate, 1.9 g fiber, 643 mg sodium*

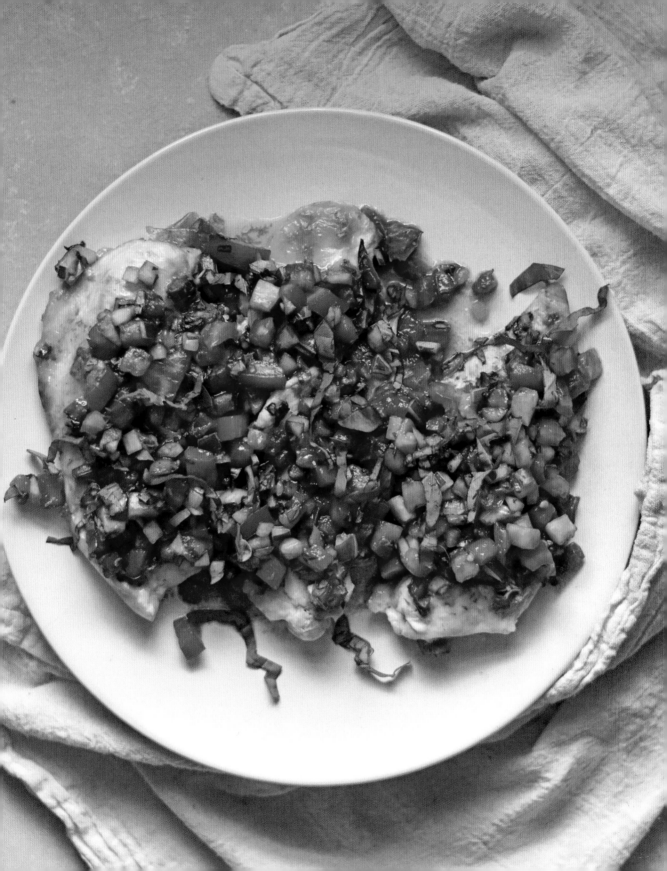

Cajun Blackened Chicken

Serves: 2 / Time: 25 minutes

INGREDIENTS

1 teaspoon garlic powder

1 teaspoon onion powder

1 teaspoon dried oregano

½ teaspoon thyme

½ teaspoon smoked paprika

¼ teaspoon cayenne

1 teaspoon sea salt

1 teaspoon freshly ground black pepper

2 tablespoons avocado oil

2 boneless, skinless chicken breasts

DIRECTIONS

In a small bowl, combine the garlic powder, onion powder, oregano, thyme, paprika, cayenne, salt, and pepper, and mix well.

In a large pan over medium heat, warm the avocado oil.

Coat each chicken breast evenly on both sides with the herb mixture. Using tongs, place the chicken in the pan.

Cover the pan and cook on each side for 10 minutes, or until the internal temperature reaches 165°F.

Serve and enjoy.

Nutrition information per serving: *313 calories, 12.9 g fat, 3.4 g saturated fat, 43.1 g protein, 4.5 g carbohydrate, 1.8 g fiber, 1,064 mg sodium*

Pesto Chicken

Serves: 4 / Time: 30 minutes

INGREDIENTS

2 tablespoons avocado oil

4 chicken breast cutlets (see Note)

¼ cup coconut flour

2 cups fresh basil leaves

¼ cup extra virgin olive oil

¼ cup pine nuts

1 teaspoon sea salt

1 garlic clove

2 tablespoons freshly grated Parmesan cheese (optional)

DIRECTIONS

Heat the avocado oil in a large skillet over medium heat.

Coat each chicken cutlet with the coconut flour and place them in the skillet. Cook for 3 to 4 minutes on each side.

Meanwhile, make the pesto. Put the basil leaves, olive oil, pine nuts, salt, and garlic in a food processor and pulse until blended. Stir in the cheese, if using.

When the chicken is almost done, pour the pesto over the chicken and cook for 3 to 5 minutes, or until the chicken is cooked through and the internal temperature reaches 165°F.

NOTE: If you can't find cutlets, simply butterfly two chicken breasts.

GIVE IT A COLLAGEN BOOST
Add 1 scoop of collagen protein to the pesto while blending.

Nutrition information per serving: *430 calories, 33.1 g fat, 6.9 g saturated fat, 13.2 g protein, 20.1 g carbohydrate, 3.8 g fiber, 997 mg sodium*

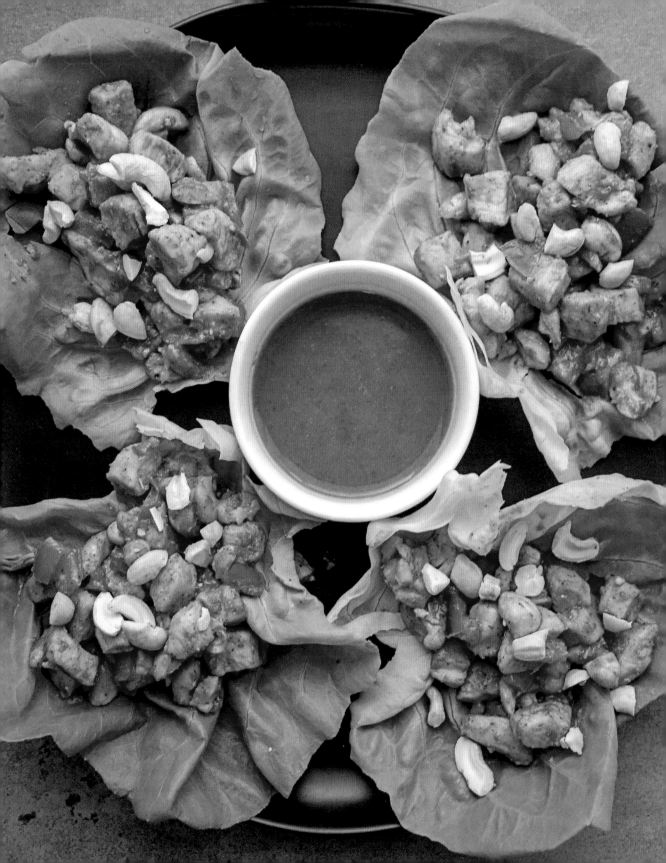

Cashew Chicken Lettuce Cups

Serves: 4 / Time: 25 minutes

INGREDIENTS

6 tablespoons coconut aminos

3 tablespoons almond butter

2 tablespoons coconut vinegar (see Note)

1 tablespoon minced fresh ginger

1 garlic clove, minced

1 teaspoon sesame oil

1 tablespoon coconut oil

1 cup diced bell peppers

1 pound boneless, skinless chicken thighs, cut into half-inch cubes

½ cup roughly chopped cashews, plus more for topping

4 butter lettuce leaves

DIRECTIONS

In a small bowl, whisk together the coconut aminos, almond butter, vinegar, ginger, garlic, and sesame oil. Set aside.

Heat the coconut oil in a large skillet over medium heat until melted. Add the bell peppers and sauté for 5 minutes, or until soft.

Add the chicken and 3 tablespoons of the sauce to the skillet and cook for 10 minutes, or until the chicken is cooked through and the liquid in the skillet evaporates.

Add the chopped cashews to the skillet and pour the remaining sauce over the chicken, veggies, and cashews. Mix well.

Place about ½ cup of the chicken mixture on each lettuce cup. Top with more cashews, if desired, and serve.

NOTE: The coconut vinegar can be replaced with 1 tablespoon white balsamic vinegar and 1 tablespoon apple cider vinegar.

MAKE IT VEGAN

Use extra-firm tofu instead of chicken.

Nutrition information per serving: *350 calories, 16.4 g fat, 4.9 g saturated fat, 36.8 g protein, 13.5 g carbohydrate, 2.4 g fiber, 103 mg sodium*

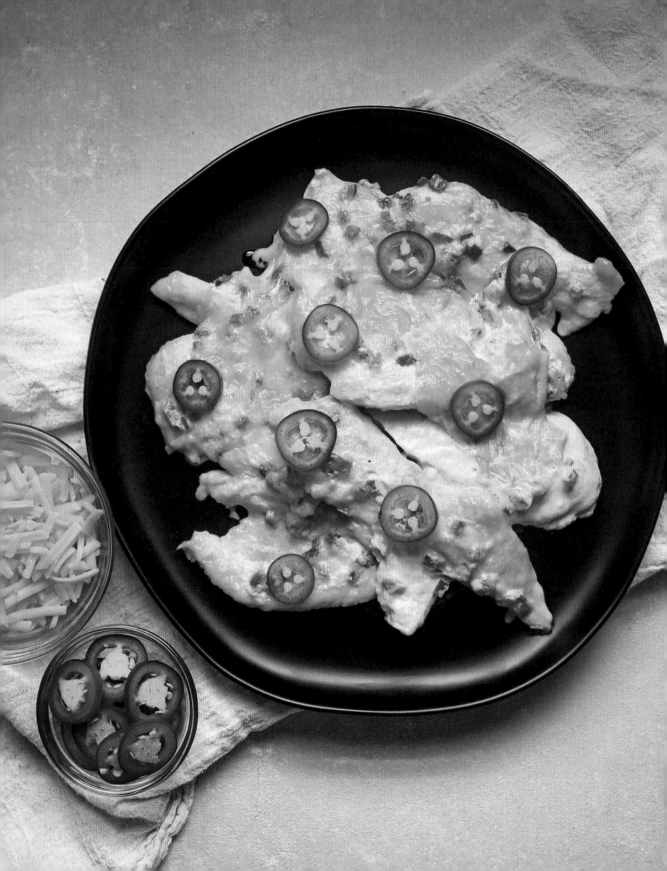

Cheesy Jalapeño Chicken

Serves: 4 / Time: 50 minutes

INGREDIENTS

6 boneless, skinless chicken breasts (1 to 1½ pounds), sliced in half lengthwise

½ teaspoon garlic powder

Pinch of sea salt

4 jalapeños

6 ounces cream cheese, softened

1 cup shredded cheddar cheese

DIRECTIONS

Preheat the oven to 375°F.

Place the chicken slices evenly in a large casserole dish and sprinkle with the garlic powder and salt.

Dice 3 of the jalapeños. In a small bowl, mix them with the cream cheese. Spread the mixture over the chicken.

Top with the cheddar. Cover the dish with foil and bake for 30 minutes.

Remove the foil and bake for 10 minutes, or until the chicken is cooked through and reaches an internal temperature of 165°F.

Thinly slice the last jalapeño and scatter it on top for a fresh kick of heat.

Nutrition information per serving: *437 calories, 28 g fat, 15.3 g saturated fat, 42.3 g protein, 2.6 g carbohydrate, 0.4 g fiber, 437 mg sodium*

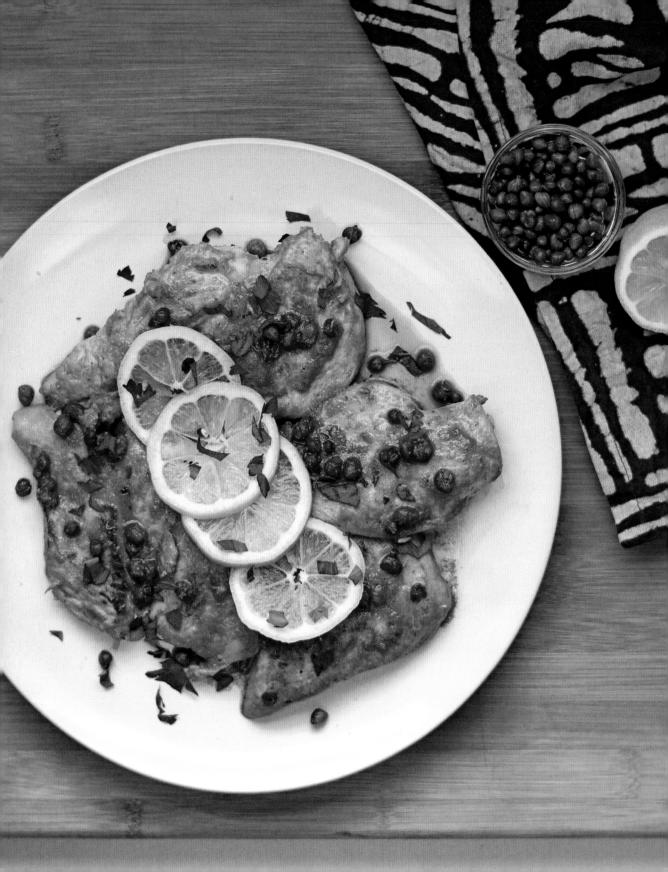

Chicken Piccata

Serves: 2 / Time: 20 minutes

INGREDIENTS

2 tablespoons grass-fed ghee or cultured butter

1 tablespoon avocado oil

2 boneless, skinless chicken breasts, sliced in half lengthwise

Juice of 1 lemon

½ cup bone broth

2 tablespoons capers

1 tablespoon coconut flour

½ teaspoon chopped parsley

Sea salt and freshly ground black pepper, to taste

DIRECTIONS

Heat a large skillet over medium heat and add the butter and avocado oil.

Add the chicken to the skillet and cook for 5 minutes on each side. Remove the chicken to a plate.

Add the lemon juice, bone broth, capers, coconut flour, parsley, salt, and pepper to the skillet. Stir constantly to prevent the coconut flour from sticking to the skillet.

Return the chicken to the skillet. Cook for 2 to 3 minutes, or until the internal temperature reaches 165°F.

Remove the chicken to a serving plate. Spoon the gravy and capers over the chicken and serve warm.

MAKE IT DAIRY FREE

Use 3 tablespoons avocado oil in place of the ghee or butter.

Nutrition information per serving: *560 calories, 24.2 g fat, 9.7 g saturated fat, 74.9 g protein, 8 g carbohydrate, 3.7 g fiber, 568 mg sodium*

Main Dishes

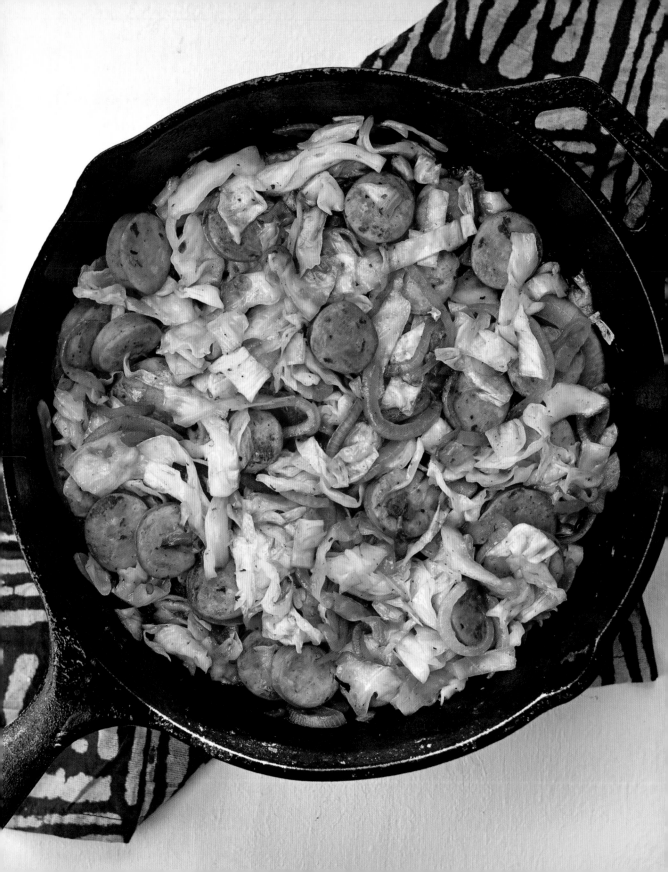

Chicken Sausage
and Cabbage

Serves: 2 / Time: 30 minutes

INGREDIENTS

1 tablespoon avocado oil

½ yellow onion, sliced

2 garlic cloves, minced

2 links organic chicken sausage (no sugar added), sliced

¼ small green cabbage, shredded

¼ cup water

Pinch of salt

DIRECTIONS

Heat a large skillet over medium heat and add the avocado oil, onion, and garlic. Sauté for 4 to 5 minutes, or until the onion is translucent.

Add the chicken sausage and cook for 3 to 4 minutes on each side.

Add the cabbage, water, and salt. Cook for 5 minutes, or until the cabbage has softened and the water has evaporated. Serve warm.

Nutrition information per serving: *207 calories, 8 g fat, 2.2 g saturated fat, 17.7 g protein, 16.1 g carbohydrate, 4.2 g fiber, 596 mg sodium*

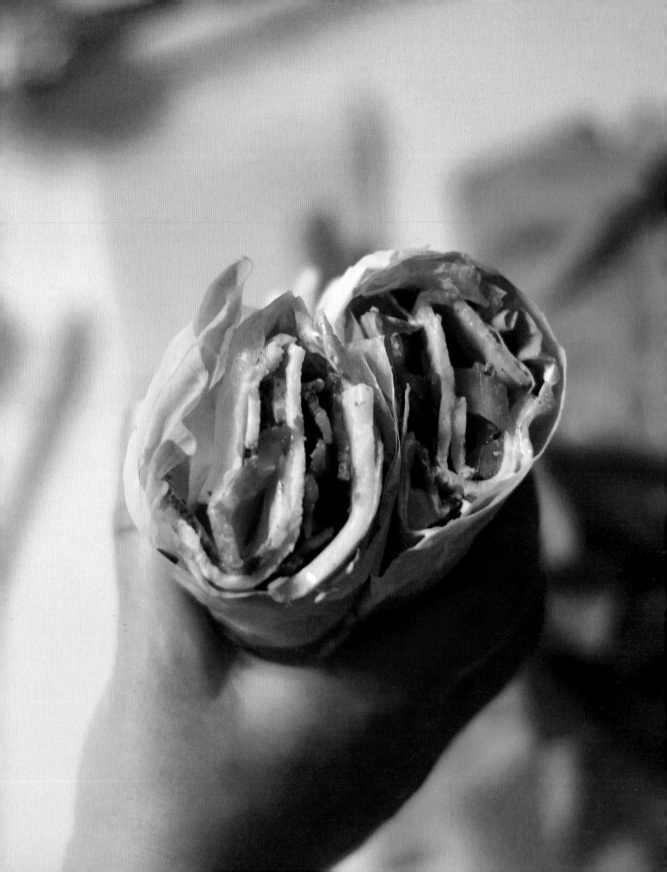

Club Sandwich Lettuce Wrap

Serves: 1 / Time: 5 minutes

INGREDIENTS

4 butter lettuce or
romaine leaves

1 tablespoon avocado oil
mayonnaise

2 slices turkey

1 slice cheddar cheese

3 slices beef or turkey
bacon, cooked

2 tomato slices

DIRECTIONS

On a piece of parchment paper, lay out the lettuce pieces as flat as possible, making a square for the butter leaves or a rectangle for the romaine leaves.

Spread the mayonnaise over the leaves and top with the turkey, cheddar, bacon, and tomatoes.

Carefully roll the sandwich up lengthwise and wrap with parchment paper to keep it secure. Cut the rolled sandwich in half. Peel back the parchment paper as you eat.

Nutrition information per serving: *372 calories, 23.3 g fat, 7.7 g saturated fat, 31.3 g protein, 5.8 g carbohydrate, 1.1 g fiber, 1,495 mg sodium*

Main Dishes

Coconut Chicken Tenders

Serves: 3 / Time: 45 minutes

INGREDIENTS

2 tablespoons coconut
oil, melted

¼ cup coconut flour

1 teaspoon sea salt

¼ teaspoon freshly ground
black pepper

¼ teaspoon garlic powder

2 large eggs, beaten

1 cup unsweetened
shredded coconut

1 pound chicken tenders

DIRECTIONS

Preheat the oven to 400°F. Place a wire rack on a parchment-lined baking sheet and brush with melted coconut oil to prevent sticking.

Arrange 3 medium bowls. In the first, put the coconut flour mixed with the sea salt, black pepper, and garlic powder; in the second, put the beaten eggs; in the third, put the shredded coconut.

Coat the chicken tenders in the coconut flour mixture, shaking off any excess. Next dredge them in the eggs, and then roll them in the shredded coconut.

Place the coated tenders on the wire rack. Avoid overcrowding. Bake for 25 minutes, or until the internal temperature reaches 165°F. Serve warm.

Nutrition information per serving: *810 calories, 57.5 g fat, 47.4 g saturated fat, 42.3 g protein, 29.9 g carbohydrate, 18.7 g fiber, 981 mg sodium*

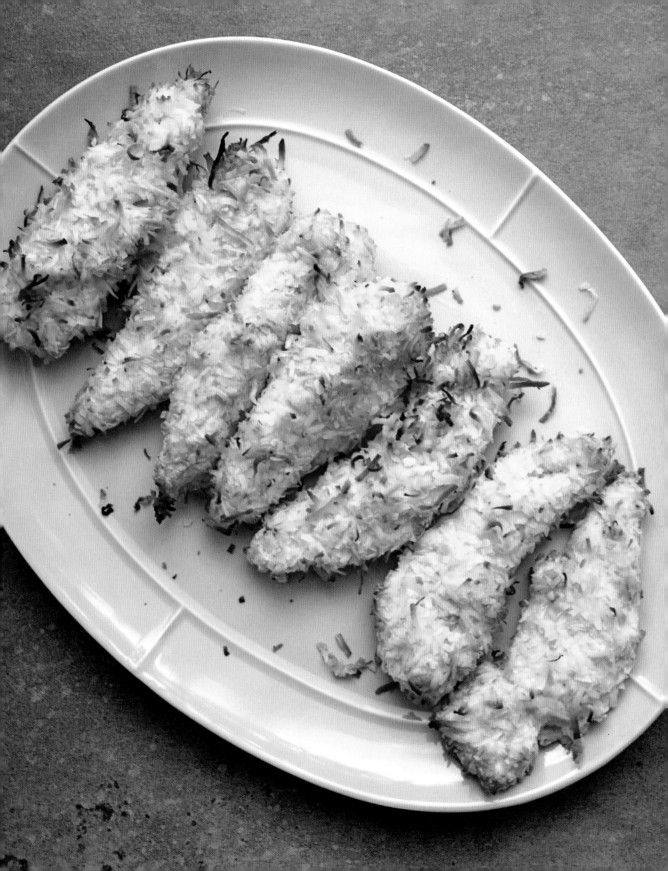

Coconut Curry and Ginger Chicken Meatballs

Serves: 4 / Time: 30 minutes

INGREDIENTS

1 pound ground chicken

1 inch fresh ginger, peeled and minced

2 garlic cloves, minced

½ teaspoon sea salt

1 tablespoon coconut aminos

2 tablespoons coconut oil

1 (4-ounce) can red Thai curry paste

1 (15-ounce) can full-fat coconut milk

DIRECTIONS

In a medium bowl, mix the ground chicken, ginger, garlic, salt, and coconut aminos. Scoop out tablespoonfuls of the meat mixture and roll into 1-inch balls. Repeat, using the rest of the meat.

Melt the coconut oil in a large skillet over medium heat and add the meatballs, leaving space in between. Cook for 8 to 10 minutes, making sure to cook the meatballs on all sides. Remove them as they are cooked to a plate.

Add the Thai curry paste to the skillet and toast for 1 minute. Pour in the coconut milk and mix together. Return the meatballs to the skillet and cook for 4 to 5 minutes. Serve warm.

Nutrition information per serving: *571 calories, 44 g fat, 30.3 g saturated fat, 35.1 g protein, 8.4 g carbohydrate, 0 g fiber, 1,403 mg sodium*

Eggplant Rollatini

Serves: 8 / Time: 1 hour

INGREDIENTS

2 large eggplants

1 teaspoon sea salt

1 teaspoon freshly ground black pepper

2 large eggs

3 cups fresh spinach

1 (4-ounce) package goat feta cheese

1 teaspoon dried oregano

1 teaspoon chopped parsley

1 teaspoon dried basil

2 cups grated Pecorino Romano, divided

1 cup grated sheep cheese, divided

1½ cups marinara sauce (no sugar added), divided

DIRECTIONS

Preheat the oven to 450°F. Line a baking sheet with parchment paper.

Trim off the ends of the eggplants and cut them lengthwise into half-inch slices.

Place the eggplant slices on the baking sheet and sprinkle with half of the salt and pepper.

Bake for 12 to 15 minutes, remove, and let cool. Reduce the heat to 400°F.

In a medium bowl, mix the eggs, spinach, feta cheese, oregano, parsley, basil, 1 cup of the Pecorino Romano, ½ cup of the sheep cheese, and the remaining salt and pepper. Mix until well combined.

In a 9 x 13-inch baking dish, pour ¾ cup of the marinara sauce.

Place ¼ cup of the cheese mixture at one end of an eggplant slice, roll it up and transfer it to the baking dish. Repeat until all the slices are rolled and in the baking dish.

Cover with the remaining ¾ cup of marinara sauce, the remaining 1 cup of Pecorino, and the remaining ½ cup of sheep cheese.

Bake for 25 minutes. Let cool for 10 minutes before serving.

Nutrition information per serving: *290 calories, 16.3 g fat, 11.5 g saturated fat, 16.2 g protein, 16.3 g carbohydrate, 6.6 g fiber, 1296 mg sodium*

Main Dishes

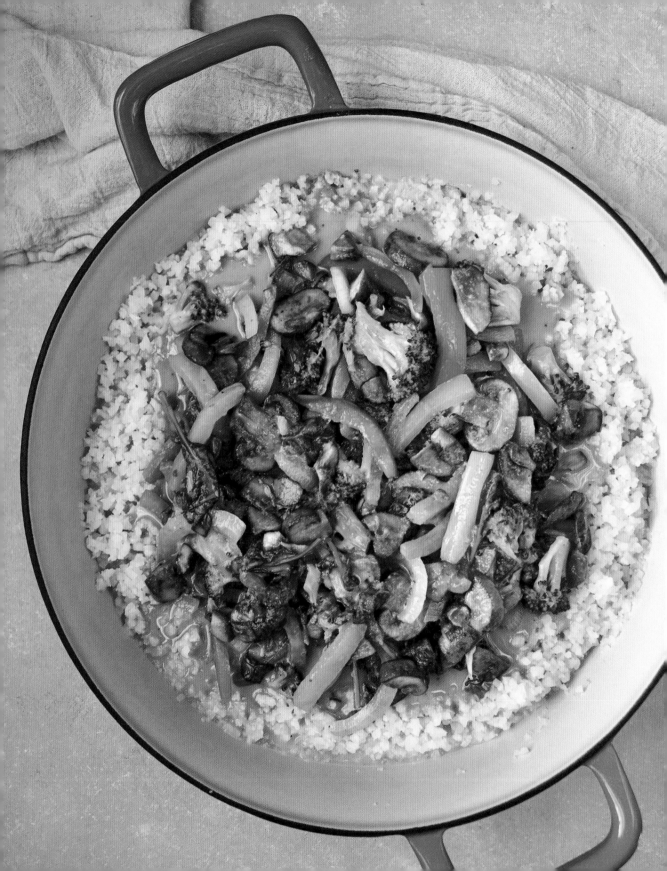

Curried Vegetables with Cauliflower Rice

Serves: 4 / Time: 25 minutes

INGREDIENTS

1 tablespoon coconut oil

1 cup broccoli florets

1 red bell pepper, sliced

1 yellow bell pepper, sliced

½ yellow onion, sliced

1 cup sliced mushrooms

1 (4-ounce) can green curry paste

1 (15-ounce) can full-fat coconut milk

1 cup fresh spinach

4 cups cooked cauliflower rice

DIRECTIONS

Melt the coconut oil in a large skillet over medium heat. Add the broccoli, bell peppers, onion, and mushrooms. Sauté for 10 minutes, or until the veggies have softened.

Push the veggies to one side of the skillet and add the green curry paste. Toast for about 30 seconds, then mix with the vegetables. Sauté for 1 minute.

Pour in the coconut milk and stir everything together. Reduce the heat to low and add the spinach. Cook until the spinach has wilted.

Serve over cauliflower rice.

Nutrition information per serving: *293 calories, 28.1 g fat, 8.4 g saturated fat, 5.8 g protein, 14 g carbohydrate, 4.8 g fiber, 314 mg sodium*

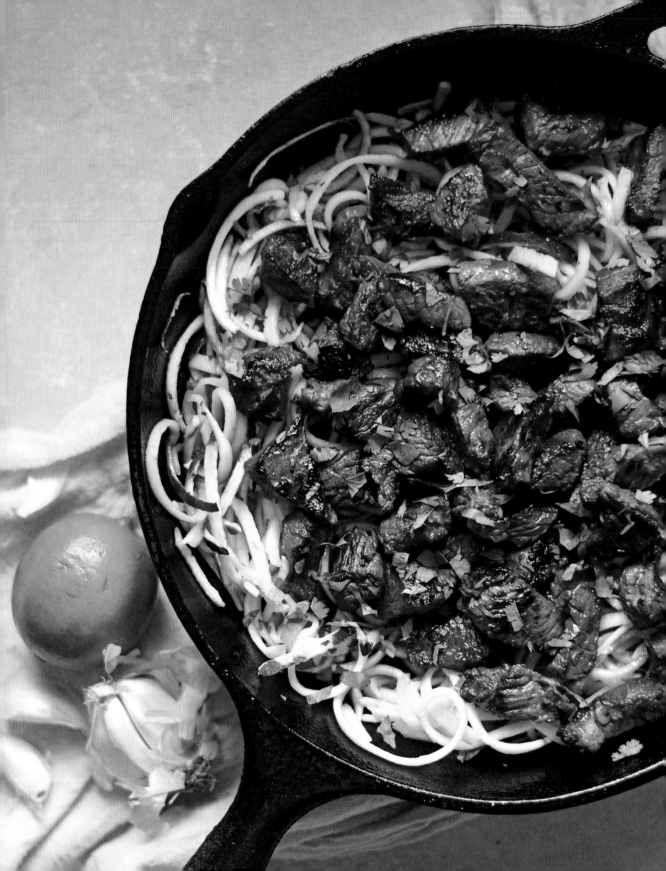

Garlic Steak Bites and Zoodles

Serves: 4 / Time: 45 minutes

INGREDIENTS

1 pound sirloin steak

¼ cup coconut aminos

1 tablespoon hot sauce

Juice of 1 lime

2 garlic cloves, minced

1 tablespoon avocado oil

3 large zucchini, spiralized into "zoodles"

Cilantro, to taste

DIRECTIONS

Cut the steak into bite-size pieces.

In a small bowl, mix together the coconut aminos, hot sauce, lime juice, and garlic. Add the steak, stir to coat completely, and let marinate for 30 minutes.

Heat a large skillet over medium-high heat and add the avocado oil. Add the meat, working in batches to avoid overcrowding the skillet.

Cook for 3 to 4 minutes, then flip the meat. Cook for 1 to 2 minutes, until all the pieces have a nice brown sear on them. Remove from the skillet to a plate.

Add the zucchini zoodles to the skillet and cook for 2 for 3 minutes, just until they have softened.

Serve the steak over the zoodles.

Nutrition information per serving: *312 calories, 18.1 g fat, 6.8 g saturated fat, 24.9 g protein, 12.8 g carbohydrate, 2.9 g fiber, 198 mg sodium*

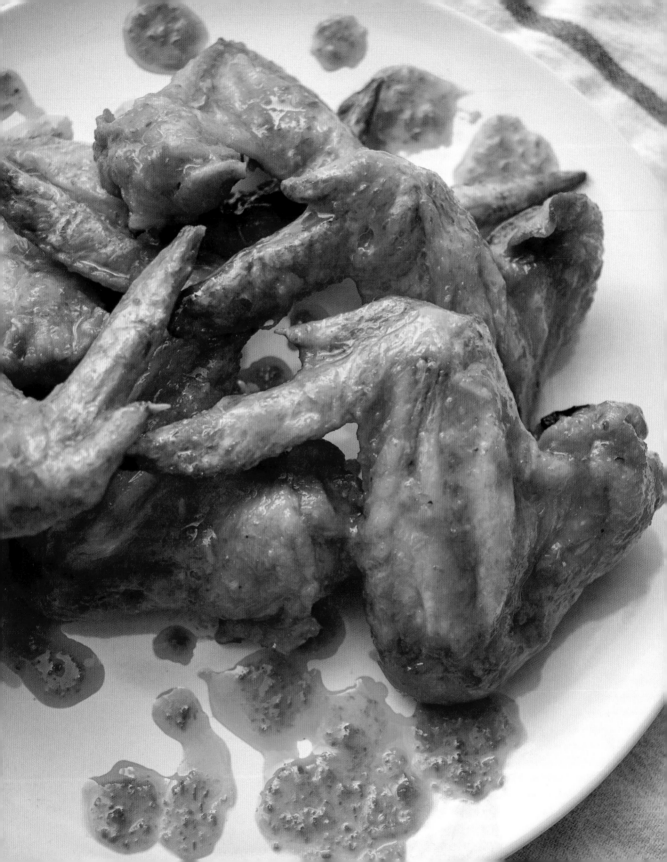

Keto Buffalo Chicken Wings

Serves: 2 / Time: 1 hour, 10 minutes

INGREDIENTS

6 whole chicken wings

1 tablespoon avocado oil

1 teaspoon sea salt

4 tablespoons grass-fed butter or ghee

¼ cup hot sauce of your choice

1 garlic clove, minced, or 1 teaspoon garlic powder

DIRECTIONS

Preheat the oven to 400°F.

In a bowl, toss the chicken wings in the avocado oil and sea salt. Set a wire rack on a baking sheet and arrange the chicken wings with space left in between them.

Bake for 20 minutes. Increase the oven temperature to 425°F and bake for 10 minutes. Be sure the chicken is cooked through and the internal temperature reaches 165°F.

In a small saucepan over medium-low heat, place the butter or ghee, hot sauce, and minced garlic and heat, stirring frequently, until the butter has melted.

Toss the chicken wings in the warm sauce and serve immediately.

Nutrition information per serving: *351 calories, 29.5 g fat, 16.9 g saturated fat, 19.4 g protein, 0.9 g carbohydrate, 0.3 g fiber, 1,698 mg sodium*

Keto Lasagna

Serves: 6 / Time: 1 hour, 30 minutes

INGREDIENTS

1 tablespoon avocado oil

½ yellow onion, diced

2 garlic cloves, minced

2 pounds ground beef

1 (32-ounce) jar marinara sauce (no sugar added)

1 teaspoon sea salt

1 large egg

1 package (15 ounces) whole-milk ricotta cheese or cashew ricotta

3 large zucchini

1 cup fresh spinach

1 cup shredded organic mozzarella cheese

DIRECTIONS

Preheat the oven to 350°F.

Heat the avocado oil in a large skillet over medium heat. Add the onion and garlic and sauté for a few minutes. Add the meat and cook for 10 minutes. Stir in the marinara sauce and salt, and mix well. Reduce the heat to low.

In a small bowl, mix the egg and ricotta together until well combined. Set aside.

Cut off the ends, and slice each zucchini lengthwise into 6 slices. Lay them out on a paper towel and pat dry.

Spread some meat sauce evenly on the bottom of a large ovenproof casserole dish.

Place the zucchini slices over the sauce in one layer, covering it. Spread half of the ricotta mixture over the zucchini slices. Top with the spinach and a little more meat sauce.

Add another layer of zucchini, followed by another layer of ricotta, spinach, and meat sauce. Continue, making 3 layers, until the sauce, spinach, and ricotta are used up.

Sprinkle the mozzarella over the top. Cover with aluminum foil and bake for 45 minutes. Remove the foil and bake for 10 to 15 minutes. Remove from the oven and let rest for at least 30 minutes before serving.

MAKE IT DAIRY FREE

Use 1 cup shredded dairy-free mozzarella, and use dairy-free ricotta in place of the whole-milk ricotta.

Nutrition information per serving: *465 calories, 20 g fat, 8.2 g saturated fat, 55.7 g protein, 15 g carbohydrate, 4.2 g fiber, 899 mg sodium*

Keto Pad Thai

Serves: 4 / Time: 35 minutes

INGREDIENTS

2 tablespoons coconut oil

1 cup snow peas

1 red pepper, sliced

½ cup sliced mushrooms

½ cup chopped red cabbage

½ cup chopped green cabbage

1 cup broccoli florets

1 cup cooked shredded chicken

3 tablespoons Thai chili sauce

1 cup full-fat coconut milk

1 zucchini, spiralized

Sauce:

1 cup cashew butter

1½ tablespoons chopped fresh ginger

⅓ cup water

⅓ cup lemon juice

4 garlic cloves, minced

1 jalapeño, stem and seeds removed

DIRECTIONS

Place a large skillet over medium-high heat until hot.

Add the coconut oil, snow peas, red pepper, mushrooms, red and green cabbage, and broccoli.

Reduce the heat to medium and sauté for 5 minutes, stirring often.

Add the chicken, Thai chili sauce, and coconut milk and continue to cook, stirring often, for 8 to 10 minutes. During the last few minutes, add the zucchini noodles.

Meanwhile, place all the sauce ingredients in a high-speed blender or food processor and blend to a saucelike consistency, adding more water if necessary.

Add the sauce to the skillet, and stir until well incorporated. Serve immediately.

Nutrition information per serving: *394 calories, 24 g fat, 9.5 g saturated fat, 21.1 g protein, 25.7 g carbohydrate, 5.1 g fiber, 481 mg sodium*

Mediterranean Grilled Lamb Chops

Serves: 2 / Time: 2 hours, 30 minutes

INGREDIENTS

4 tablespoons avocado oil

2 tablespoons lemon juice

6 garlic cloves, minced

½ teaspoon fresh thyme

2 teaspoons fresh rosemary

5 basil leaves, cut into chiffonade

¼ teaspoon nutmeg

½ teaspoon cinnamon

½ teaspoon coriander

Sea salt and freshly ground black pepper, to taste

6 lamb chops

DIRECTIONS

In a large bowl, combine the avocado oil, lemon juice, garlic, thyme, rosemary, basil, nutmeg, cinnamon, coriander, and salt and pepper for the marinade.

Add the lamb chops to the bowl and stir to coat them completely. Marinate the lamb in the refrigerator for at least 2 hours.

Remove from the refrigerator and let the lamb come to room temperature. Preheat the grill.

Place the lamb chops on the grill. Carefully spoon the marinade over the lamb chops to keep them moist while grilling.

Grill the lamb chops for 4 to 6 minutes on each side for medium-rare.

Serve and enjoy.

Nutrition information per serving: *634 calories, 25.1 g fat, 1.1 g saturated fat, 89.4 g protein, 6.5 g carbohydrate, 2.5 g fiber, 241 mg sodium*

Pecorino Mushroom Chicken

Serves: 4 / Time: 35 minutes

INGREDIENTS

¼ **cup ghee**

1 **pound mushrooms, chopped**

1 **medium yellow onion, chopped**

½ **cup chopped parsley**

¼ **cup lemon juice**

4 **garlic cloves, chopped**

Sea salt and freshly ground black pepper, to taste

4 **bone-in, skin-on chicken breasts**

¼ **cup avocado oil mayonnaise**

⅓ **cup grated Pecorino Romano**

DIRECTIONS

Preheat the oven to 500°F. Line a baking sheet with parchment paper.

Heat the ghee in a skillet over medium high-heat. Add the mushrooms, onion, parsley, lemon juice, garlic, salt, and pepper and sauté for 20 minutes, or until the mushrooms are soft. Remove the vegetables from the skillet to a bowl and set aside.

Season the chicken breasts with salt and pepper. Spread the mayonnaise over them and sprinkle them with the Pecorino Romano.

Bake the chicken for 5 minutes. Increase the oven temperature to broil and broil the chicken for 6 to 9 minutes, or until it is cooked through (the internal temperature reaches 165 degrees).

Put the chicken breasts on plates, top with the mushroom mixture, and serve.

Nutrition information per serving: *409 calories, 29.5 g fat, 11.9 g saturated fat, 28 g protein, 8.1 g carbohydrate, 2.1 g fiber, 432 mg sodium*

Main Dishes

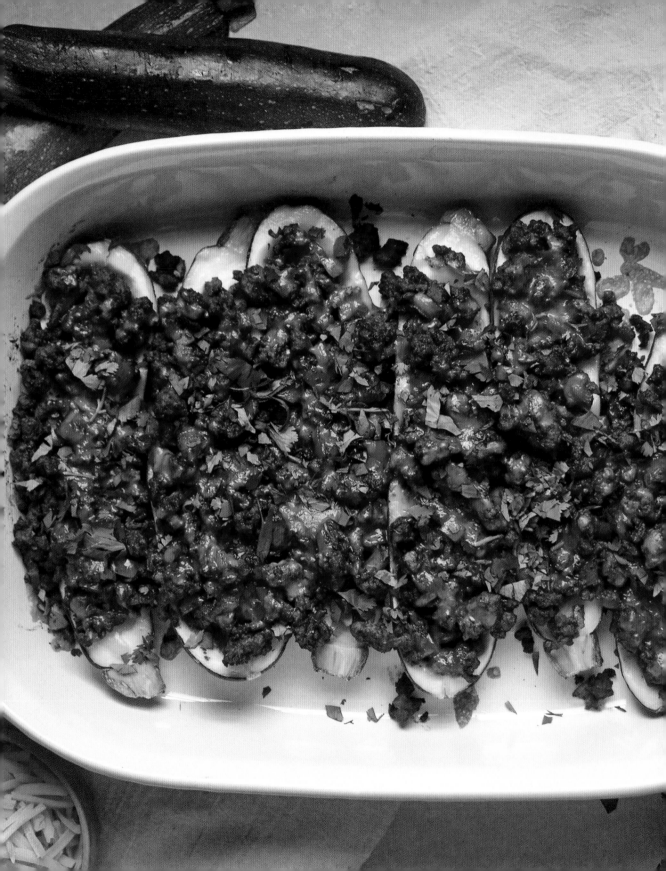

Mexican
Turkey Zucchini Boats

Serves: 4 / Time: 30 minutes

INGREDIENTS

4 medium zucchini

2 tablespoons avocado oil

½ yellow onion, diced

1 red bell pepper, diced

2 garlic cloves, minced

1 pound ground turkey

2 tablespoons tomato paste

2 tablespoons chili powder

1 tablespoon ground cumin

Sea salt and freshly ground black pepper, to taste

1 cup shredded organic cheddar cheese (optional)

1 cup fresh cilantro, chopped

DIRECTIONS

Preheat the oven to 375°F. Lightly grease a large casserole dish.

Slice the zucchini in half lengthwise and scoop out the seeds. Rub the inside of the zucchini boats with 1 tablespoon of the avocado oil. Place them in the casserole dish and bake for 15 minutes.

Meanwhile, add the remaining tablespoon of avocado oil to a large skillet over medium heat. Sauté the onion, bell pepper, and garlic for 4 to 5 minutes.

Add the ground turkey and cook for 7 to 8 minutes, or until the meat is cooked through. Stir in the tomato paste, chili powder, cumin, salt, and pepper.

Remove the mixture from the heat and spoon it into the zucchini boats. Top with the cheddar, if using, and return the zucchini to the oven for 5 to 7 minutes, or until the cheese is melted.

Top the zucchini with the cilantro and serve.

Nutrition information per serving: *418 calories, 24.2 g fat, 8.4 g saturated fat, 42.2 g protein, 15.7 g carbohydrate, 5.1 g fiber, 466 mg sodium*

Main Dishes

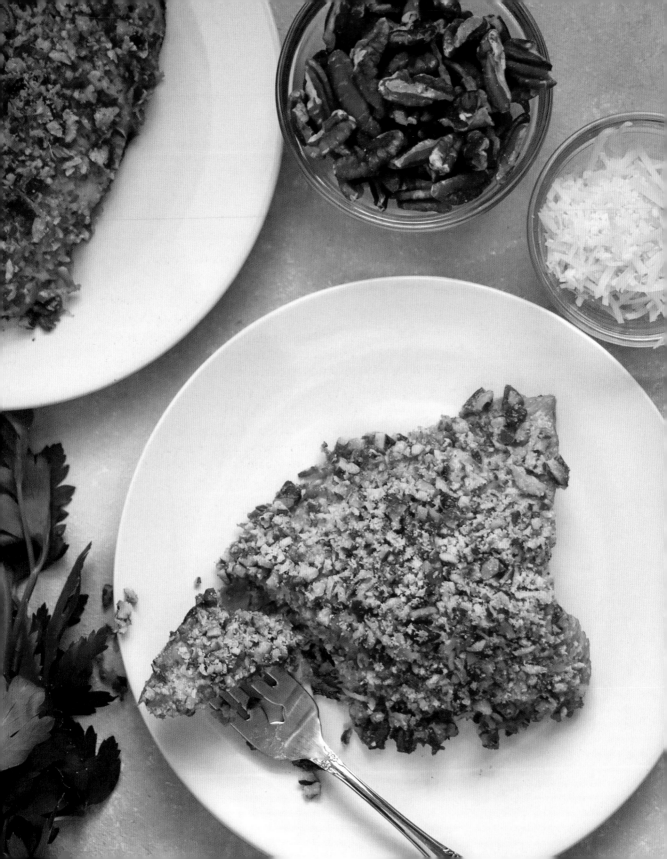

Pecan-Crusted Salmon

Serves: 2 / Time: 20 minutes

INGREDIENTS

2 tablespoons avocado oil

½ cup finely chopped
raw pecans

2 tablespoons almond flour

2 tablespoons freshly grated
Parmesan cheese

½ teaspoon sea salt

Two 6-ounce wild-caught
Alaskan salmon fillets

DIRECTIONS

Preheat the oven to 425°F. Line a baking sheet with parchment paper.

In a small bowl, mix together 1 tablespoon of the avocado oil with the pecans, almond flour, Parmesan, and salt.

Place the salmon fillets on the baking sheet. Spread the remaining 1 tablespoon of avocado oil over each salmon fillet. Top with the pecan mixture.

Bake for 12 to 15 minutes, or until the salmon is cooked through and flakes easily.

Nutrition information per serving: *410 calories, 29.8 g fat, 3.5 g saturated fat, 32.7 g protein, 5.2 g carbohydrate, 3.8 g fiber, 543 mg sodium*

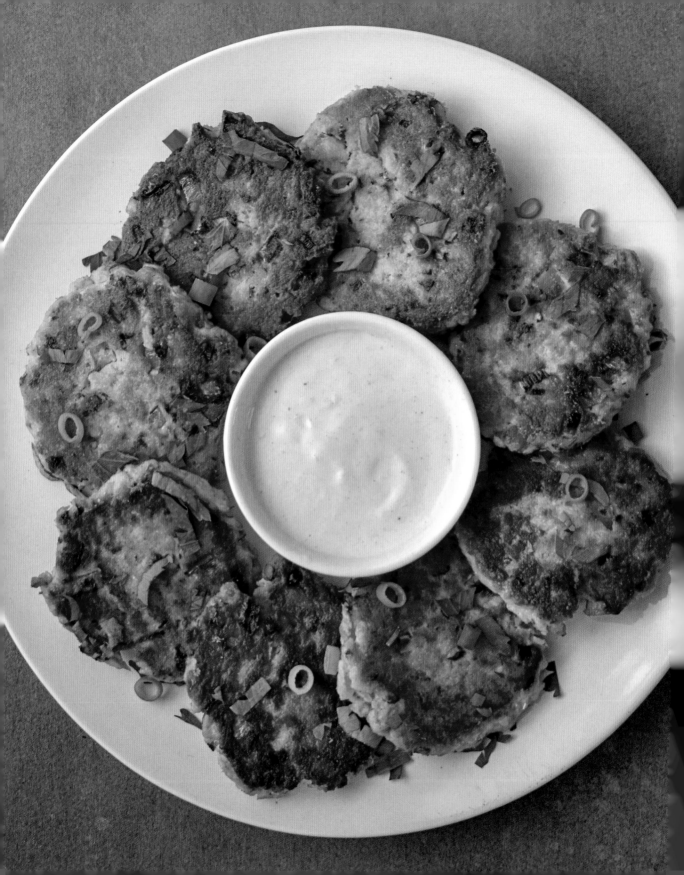

Salmon Cakes
with Garlic Aioli

Serves: 8 / Time: 15 minutes

INGREDIENTS

Salmon cakes:

2 (6-ounce) cans wild-caught salmon

1 tablespoon avocado oil mayonnaise

2 green onions, chopped

½ small bell pepper, diced

¼ cup finely chopped fresh Italian parsley or dill

¼ cup almond flour

2 large eggs

Pinch of sea salt

2 tablespoons avocado oil

Garlic aioli:

¼ cup avocado oil mayonnaise

½ tablespoon Dijon mustard

½ tablespoon lemon juice

1 garlic clove, minced

DIRECTIONS

In a medium bowl, mix together the salmon, mayonnaise, green onions, bell pepper, parsley, almond flour, eggs, and salt.

With clean hands, form eight round patties, about ½ inch thick.

Heat the oil in a large skillet over medium-high heat and carefully add the patties.

Cook each patty for 4 minutes, then flip and cook for 3 to 4 minutes.

In a small bowl, whisk together the aioli ingredients. Pour into a small ramekin and serve with the patties.

GIVE IT A COLLAGEN BOOST:

Add 1 scoop of collagen protein to the salmon mixture before forming the patties.

Nutrition information per serving: *115 calories, 9.3 g fat, 1.7 g saturated fat, 5.1 g protein, 2.3 g carbohydrate, 0.7 g fiber, 179 mg sodium*

Sautéed Pesto Mahi Mahi

Serves: 4 / Time: 15 minutes

INGREDIENTS

½ cup fresh basil, lightly packed

½ cup fresh sage, lightly packed

½ cup fresh cilantro, lightly packed

½ cup fresh parsley, lightly packed

2 garlic cloves

½ cup extra virgin olive oil

¼ cup pine nuts

½ cup freshly grated Parmesan cheese

1 tablespoon coconut oil

4 wild-caught mahi mahi fish fillets (appoximately 6 ounces each)

1 lemon, halved

DIRECTIONS

Combine the basil, sage, cilantro, parsley, garlic, oil, and pine nuts in a food processor, and process until the mixture is creamy. Pulse in the Parmesan.

Heat the coconut oil in a large skillet over medium-high heat until it just starts to smoke.

Spread the pesto on both sides of the fish fillets. Sauté the fish in the skillet until it flakes easily, 3 to 5 minutes per side.

When the fish is done, brush both sides with pesto again. Squeeze the lemon over the fish and serve immediately.

Nutrition information per serving: *511 calories, 40.7 g fat, 10 g saturated fat, 36.8 g protein, 3.5 g carbohydrate, 0.9 g fiber, 239 mg sodium*

Steak Fajitas

Serves: 8 / Time: 8 hours

INGREDIENTS

Fajitas:

1½ pounds skirt steak, cut into thin strips

1 green bell pepper, sliced

1 red bell pepper, sliced

1 red onion, sliced

2 jalapeños, sliced

2 cups salsa

1 tablespoon chili powder

1 tablespoon dried oregano

1 tablespoon cumin

1 tablespoon garlic powder

½ tablespoon onion powder

1 teaspoon smoked paprika

1 teaspoon sea salt

1 teaspoon freshly ground black pepper

8 almond flour tortillas

Toppings (optional):

Finely chopped kale

Plain goat yogurt

Tomatoes, chopped

Green onions, chopped

Cilantro, to taste

DIRECTIONS

Place the steak, vegetables and all the seasonings into a crockpot and cook on low for 8 hours.

Serve on the tortillas with the kale, goat yogurt, tomatoes, green onions, and cilantro, as desired.

Nutrition information per serving: *283 calories, 10.2 g fat, 3.7 g saturated fat, 27 g protein, 22.2 g carbohydrate, 4.9 g fiber, 725 mg sodium*

Shepherd's Pie

Serves: 6 / Time: 1 hour

INGREDIENTS

1 tablespoon avocado oil

½ yellow onion, diced

3 celery stalks, diced

1 pound ground beef

2 cups cauliflower, chopped

¼ cup unsweetened almond milk

2 tablespoons butter

½ teaspoon sea salt

¼ cup tomato paste

¼ cup water

1 teaspoon dried thyme

1 teaspoon dried oregano

1 teaspoon sea salt

¼ cup peas, fresh or frozen

1 cup freshly grated Parmesan cheese

DIRECTIONS

Preheat the oven to 375°F.

Heat the avocado oil in a large skillet over medium heat. Add the onion and celery and sauté for 4 to 5 minutes. Add the ground beef and cook for 7 to 8 minutes, or until browned and cooked through.

Meanwhile, place the cauliflower in a large pot and cover with water. Bring to a boil and simmer for about 10 minutes, until fork-tender. Drain and mash the cauliflower in a bowl. Add the almond milk, butter, and sea salt, and stir. Set the cauliflower aside.

Stir into the meat and vegetable mixture the tomato paste, water, thyme, oregano, and salt. Simmer for about 10 minutes, or until the water has evaporated.

Stir in the peas and transfer the meat and vegetables to an ovenproof dish or a cast-iron skillet.

Top with the mashed cauliflower, pressing the cauliflower against the side of the dish to seal in the filling.

Top with the Parmesan, if desired, and bake for 30 minutes. Serve warm.

MAKE IT DAIRY FREE

Use coconut oil in place of butter and omit the cheese or use a dairy-free cheese instead.

Nutrition information per serving: *270 calories, 13.3 g fat, 7.2 g saturated fat, 30.7 g protein, 6.9 g carbohydrate, 2.2 g fiber, 375 mg sodium*

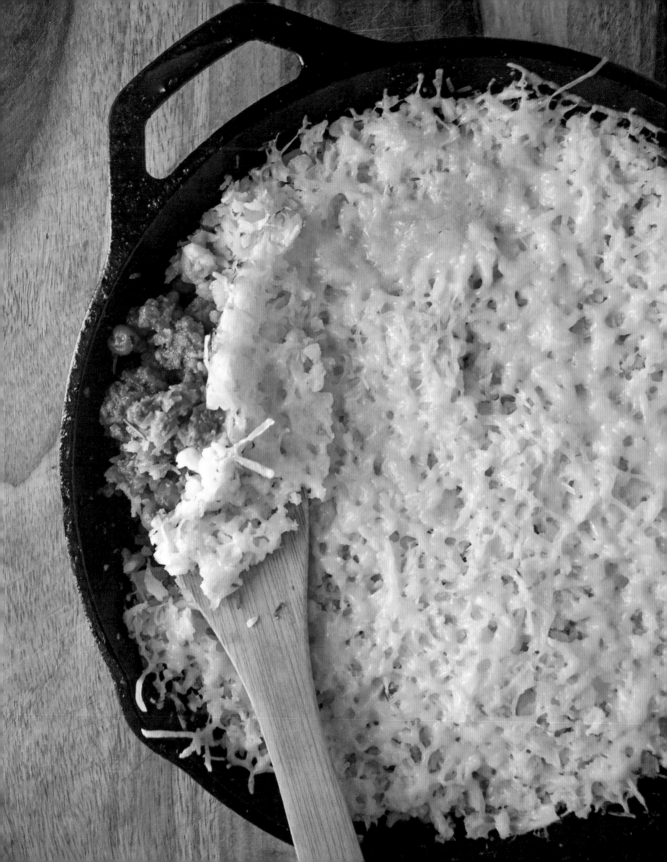

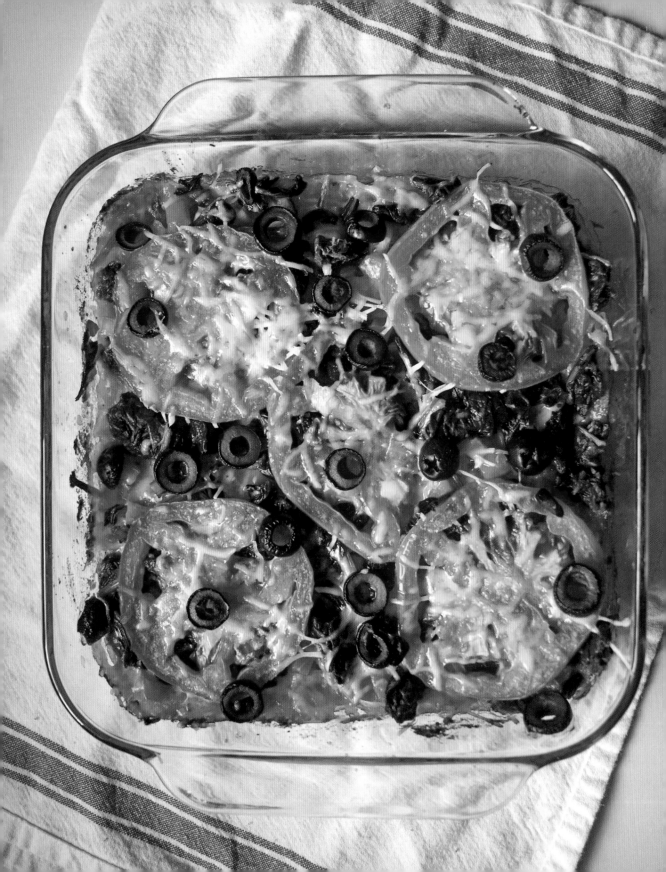

Spaghetti Squash Veggie "Pizza"

Serves: 4 / Time: 30 minutes

INGREDIENTS

1 large spaghetti squash, cooked

1 cup marinara sauce (no sugar added)

1 cup organic shredded mozzarella cheese

1 large tomato, sliced thin

1 red bell pepper, diced

1 cup frozen spinach

¼ cup sliced black olives

DIRECTIONS

Preheat the oven to 400°F.

Shred the cooked spaghetti squash and place in a colander over a large bowl or in the sink. Let it drain for 10 minutes.

In a medium bowl, stir the marinara sauce and the spaghetti squash together. Pour the mixture into an 8 x 8-inch casserole dish and press it down.

Top with the cheese, tomato, bell pepper, spinach, and black olives. Bake for 20 minutes.

Divide onto four plates and serve immediately.

MAKE IT VEGAN AND DAIRY FREE
Use a nut-based "mozzarella" cheese.

Nutrition information per serving: *255 calories, 4 g fat, 1.3 g saturated fat, 7.8 g protein, 13.7 g carbohydrate, 10.9 g fiber, 482 mg sodium*

Thai Curry Kelp Noodles

Serves: 6 / Time: 20 minutes

INGREDIENTS

Curry sauce:

2 tablespoons hot water

2 tablespoons nut butter of choice

2 teaspoons red curry paste

Juice of ½ lime

Kelp noodles:

1 tablespoon coconut oil

1½ cups broccoli florets

2 packages kelp noodles, rinsed and drained

1 tablespoon coconut aminos

1 cup kimchi

DIRECTIONS

In a medium mixing bowl, combine the hot water, nut butter, curry paste, and lime juice, stirring until well blended. Set aside.

Melt the coconut oil in a cast-iron skillet over medium heat.

When the skillet is hot, add the broccoli florets. Sauté for 5 to 7 minutes, or until tender.

Remove the skillet from the heat and add the kelp noodles and coconut aminos, stirring until well combined.

Transfer the noodle mixture to a medium bowl and top with the kimchi.

Drizzle the curry sauce over and serve.

Nutrition information per serving: *171 calories, 8.1 g fat, 3.1 g saturated fat, 3.7 g protein, 20.2 g carbohydrate, 9.5 g fiber, 786 mg sodium*

Turkey-Stuffed Bell Peppers

Serves: 4 / Time: 1 hour, 10 minutes

INGREDIENTS

1 tablespoon avocado oil

1 pound ground turkey

3 garlic cloves, minced

¼ red onion, minced

¼ cup chopped parsley

½ teaspoon sea salt

½ teaspoon freshly ground black pepper

1 cup marinara sauce (no sugar added)

½ cup riced cauliflower

4 large bell peppers of choice, halved lengthwise, stems and seeds removed

Crumbled goat feta cheese, to taste

DIRECTIONS

Preheat the oven to 375°F. Grease an 8 x 8-inch baking dish.

Put the oil in a large skillet over medium heat.

Add the turkey and cook for about 3 minutes, keeping it still pink.

Add the garlic, onion, parsley, salt, and pepper to the turkey and cook until the turkey is done, 3 to 5 minutes.

Remove from the heat and add the marinara sauce and riced cauliflower.

Place the bell peppers cut-side up in the baking dish and fill them with the turkey mixture.

Sprinkle with the feta cheese and bake for 45 minutes.

Remove from the oven and serve.

Nutrition information per serving: *377 calories, 19.9 g fat, 6.2 g saturated fat, 38 g protein, 16.6 g carbohydrate, 4.3 g fiber, 671 mg sodium*

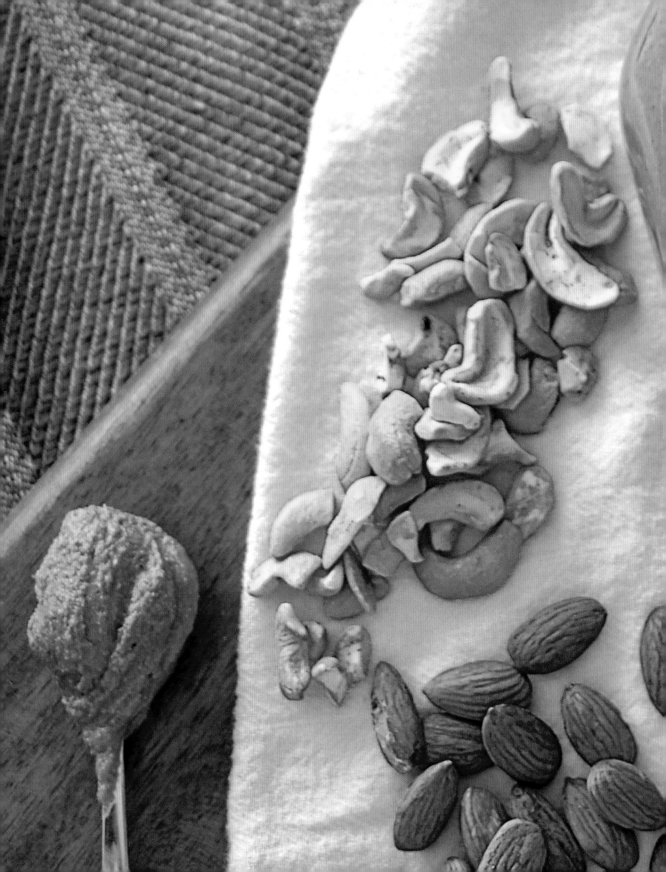

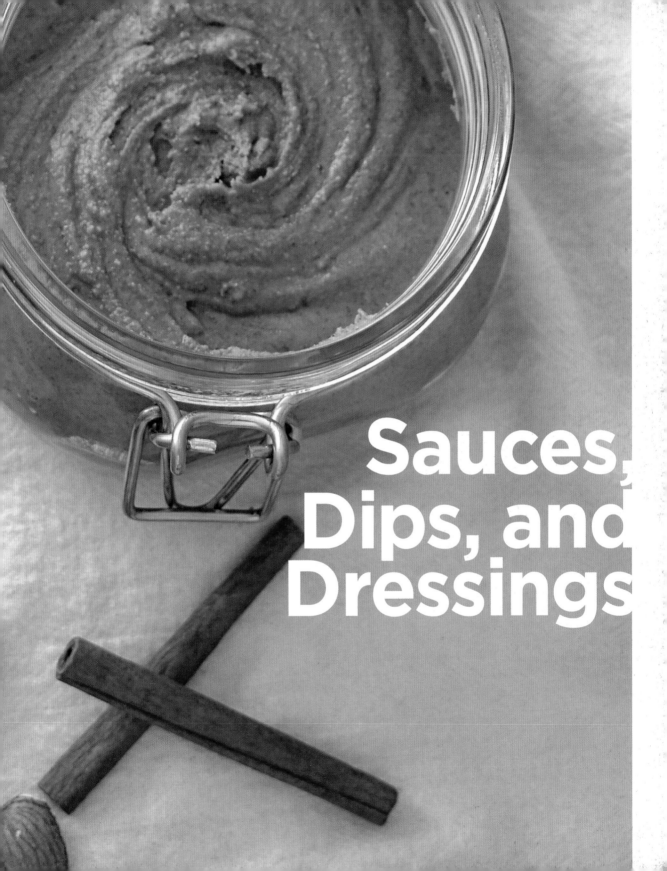

Sauces, Dips, and Dressings

Artichoke Dip

Serves: 3 / Time: 15 minutes

INGREDIENTS

1 (14-ounce) can artichoke hearts, drained

1 pound goat cheese (chèvre)

2 tablespoons extra virgin olive oil

2 teaspoons lemon juice

1 garlic clove, minced

1 tablespoon chopped parsley

1 tablespoon chopped chives

½ tablespoon chopped basil

½ teaspoon sea salt

½ teaspoon freshly ground black pepper

Dash of cayenne pepper (optional)

½ cup freshly grated Pecorino Romano

DIRECTIONS

In a food processor, combine all the ingredients, except the Pecorino Romano, and process until well incorporated and creamy.

Top with the freshly grated Pecorino Romano. Store in an airtight container in the refrigerator for up to 3 days.

Nutrition information per serving: *455 calories, 36.1 g fat, 19.4 g saturated fat, 21.9 g protein, 13.3 g carbohydrate, 2.3 g fiber, 1,728 mg sodium*

Avocado
Ranch Dressing

Serves: 4 / Time: 15 minutes

INGREDIENTS

1 cup sour cream

2 tablespoons chopped green onions

2 teaspoons chopped fresh thyme

2 teaspoons chopped fresh parsley

1 teaspoon chopped fresh dill

2 teaspoons roasted garlic purée (homemade or store-bought)

¼ teaspoon onion powder

¼ teaspoon paprika

⅛ teaspoon cayenne pepper

Sea salt and freshly ground black pepper, to taste

2 avocados

DIRECTIONS

Combine all the ingredients in a food processor and process until smooth and creamy. Store in an airtight container in the refrigerator for up to 3 days.

Nutrition information per serving: *334 calories, 31.7 g fat, 11.6 g saturated fat, 4 g protein, 12.5 g carbohydrate, 7.1 g fiber, 97 mg sodium*

Cashew Caesar Dressing

Serves: 4 / Time: 5 minutes

INGREDIENTS

½ cup raw cashews, soaked for at least 6 hours

Juice of ½ lemon

3 oil-packed anchovy fillets

2 teaspoons Dijon mustard

2 garlic cloves, minced

½ teaspoon sea salt

2 tablespoons extra virgin olive oil

⅓ cup water

DIRECTIONS

Combine all the ingredients, except the water, in a high-speed blender. Blend, gradually adding the water until the dressing reaches the desired consistency. Store in an airtight container in the refrigerator for up to 3 days.

MAKE IT VEGAN

Replace the anchovies with 2 teaspoons capers.

GIVE IT A COLLAGEN BOOST

Add 1 scoop of collagen protein before blending.

Nutrition information per serving: *457 calories, 42.5 g fat, 5.8 g saturated fat, 13.4 g protein, 10.1 g carbohydrate, 1.1 g fiber, 3,753 mg sodium*

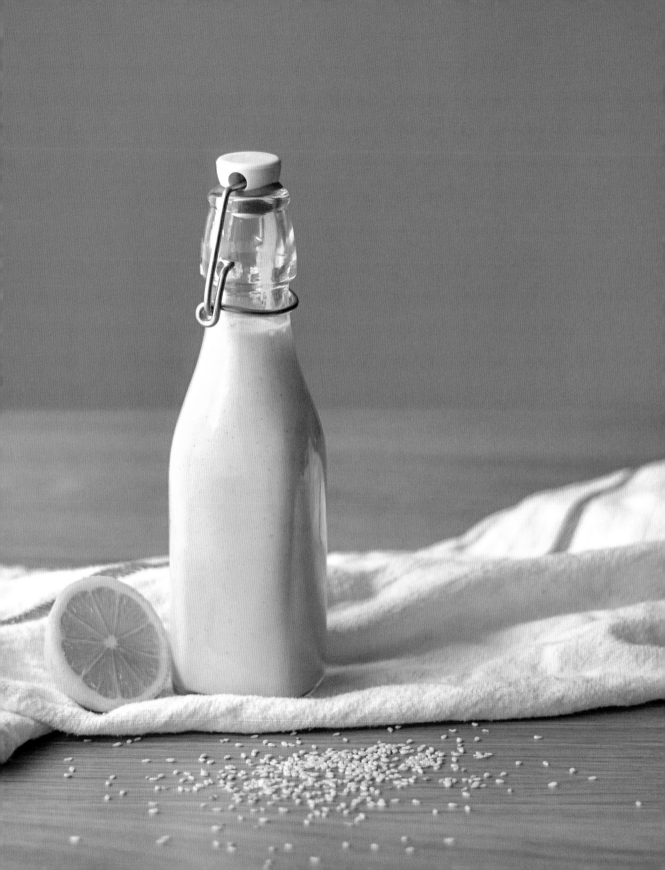

Chimichurri

Serves: 4 / Time: 5 minutes

INGREDIENTS

½ cup extra virgin olive oil

Juice of 3 limes

1 red pepper, chopped

1 red chili pepper, chopped

2 shallots, chopped

2 Roma tomatoes, chopped

½ red onion, chopped

4 to 5 garlic cloves, chopped

½ bunch parsley

½ bunch cilantro

½ teaspoon sea salt

½ teaspoon thyme

½ teaspoon chili powder

½ teaspoon smoked paprika

DIRECTIONS

Place all the ingredients in a food processor and process until well combined. Store in an airtight container in the refrigerator for up to 3 days.

Nutrition information per serving: *296 calories, 26.1 g fat, 3.7 g saturated fat, 4.1 g protein, 17.6 g carbohydrate, 4.6 g fiber, 290 mg sodium*

Dijon Vinaigrette

Serves: 8 / Time: 5 minutes

INGREDIENTS

¼ cup extra virgin olive oil

¼ cup white balsamic vinegar

2 tablespoons Dijon mustard

¼ teaspoon garlic powder

Pinch of salt

1 teaspoon monk fruit syrup, maple flavored (optional)

DIRECTIONS

In a small bowl, whisk all the ingredients together until the mustard is blended in fully. Store in an airtight container in a cool spot on the counter for 3 to 4 days or in the refrigerator for a week.

Nutrition information per serving: *468 calories, 51.7 g fat, 7.3 g saturated fat, 1.5 g protein, 2.7 g carbohydrate, 1.1 g fiber, 513 mg sodium*

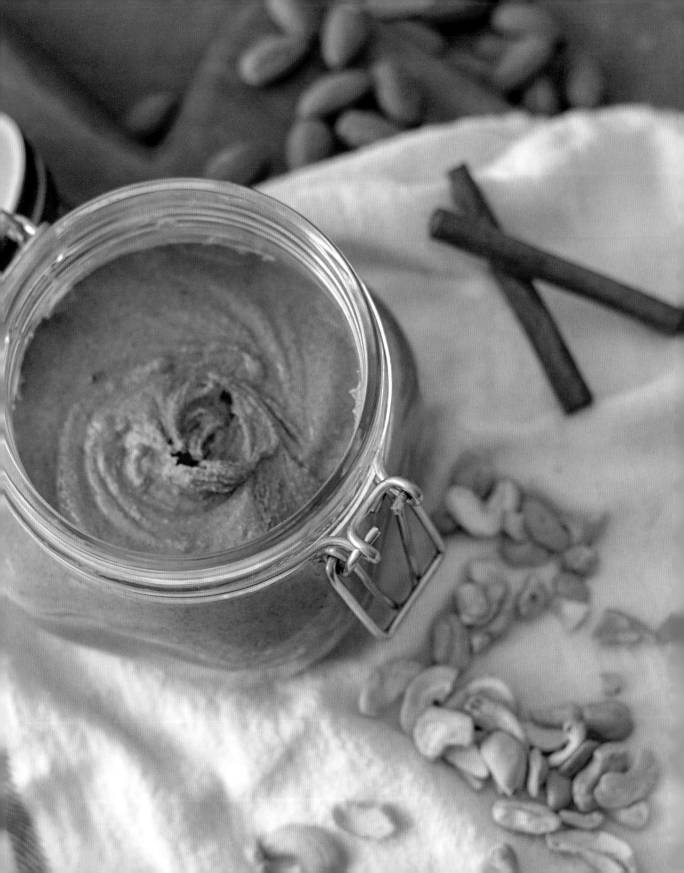

Cinnamon Nut Butter

Serves: 20 / Time: 15 minutes

INGREDIENTS

1½ cups dry-roasted, unsalted almonds

1½ cups dry-roasted, unsalted cashews

2 tablespoons nut oil (macadamia, almond, or cashew)

1 tablespoon cinnamon or pumpkin pie spice

¼ teaspoon sea salt

1 teaspoon pure vanilla extract

DIRECTIONS

Combine all the ingredients in a high-speed blender. Blend for 10 minutes or longer, or until creamy. Store in an airtight container in the refrigerator for up to 2 weeks or in the freezer for up to 4 months.

GIVE IT A COLLAGEN BOOST

Add 1 scoop of collagen protein before blending.

Nutrition information per serving: *809 calories, 72.3 g fat, 8.3 g saturated fat, 18.3 g protein, 28.5 g carbohydrate, 11.1 g fiber, 469 mg sodium*

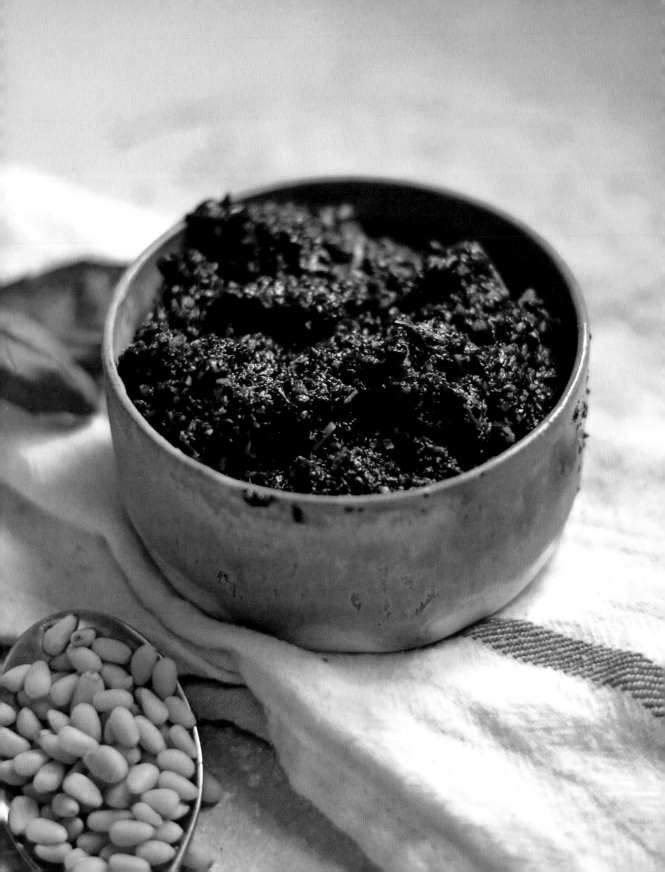

Kale Pesto

Serves: 4 / Time: 5 minutes

INGREDIENTS

1 bunch curly kale (about 2 cups), stemmed

1 bunch fresh basil (about 1 cup), stemmed

2 garlic cloves

2 tablespoons pine nuts or slivered almonds

2 tablespoons freshly grated Parmesan cheese (optional)

¼ cup plus 2 tablespoons extra virgin olive oil

DIRECTIONS

Add all the ingredients, except the olive oil, to a food processor or a high-speed blender.

With the processor running, slowly drizzle in the olive oil. Blend until everything is well incorporated. Store in an airtight container in the refrigerator for up to 1 week.

Nutrition information per serving: *280 calories, 31.1 g fat, 4.2 g saturated fat, 1.3 g protein, 2.8 g carbohydrate, 0.8 g fiber, 7 mg sodium*

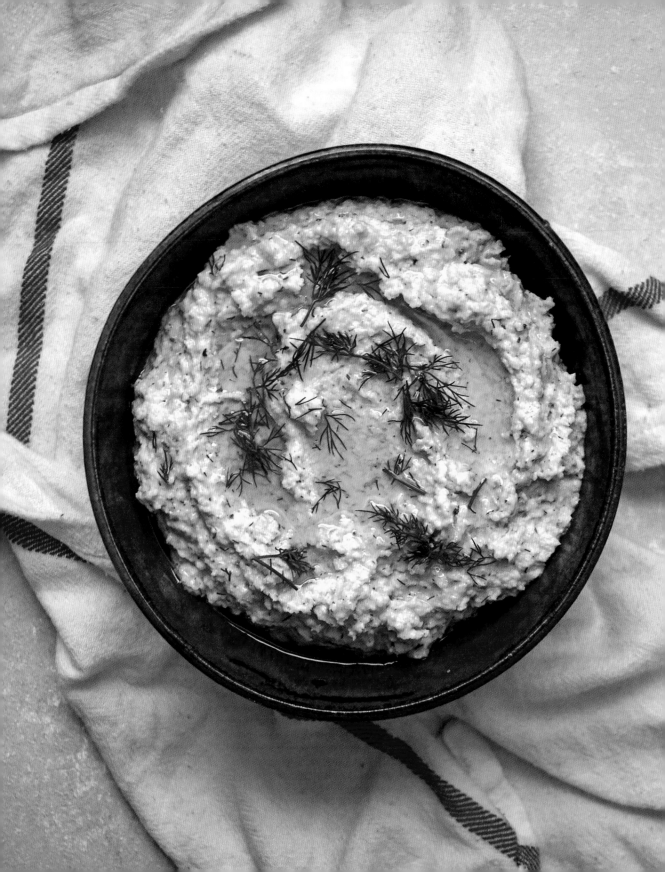

Roasted Cauliflower Dill Dip

Serves: 8 / Time: 50 minutes

INGREDIENTS

1 small cauliflower

2 garlic cloves

2 tablespoons extra virgin olive oil, plus additional as needed

½ shallot

¼ cup tahini

¼ cup extra virgin olive oil

2 ounces cream cheese

¼ cup fresh dill, stemmed

Pinch of salt

DIRECTIONS

Preheat the oven to 425°F.

Remove the leaves and large stem, then chop the cauliflower.

Place the cauliflower and garlic cloves on a baking sheet and toss with the olive oil. Roast for 20 to 25 minutes, tossing halfway through. Remove from the oven and let cool.

Place the vegetables in a food processor or high-speed blender. Add the remaining ingredients and pulse until it forms a dip consistency. Add additional olive oil 1 tablespoon at a time if a thinner consistency is desired.

Store in an airtight container in the refrigerator for 3 to 4 days.

MAKE IT DAIRY FREE

Use a nut-based cream cheese instead of dairy cream cheese.

Nutrition information per serving: *169 calories, 17.1 g fat, 3.6 g saturated fat, 2.4 g protein, 3.9 g carbohydrate, 1.1 g fiber, 55 mg sodium*

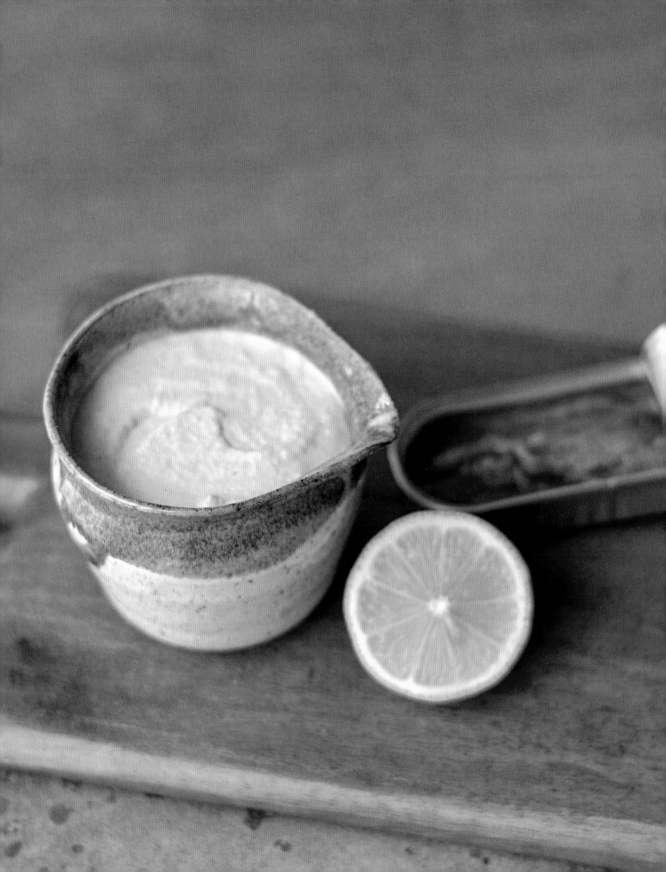

Tahini Lemon Dressing

Serves: 4 / Time: 5 minutes

INGREDIENTS

½ cup tahini

Juice of 1 large lemon

2 tablespoons extra virgin olive oil

1 teaspoon sea salt

1 teaspoon Dijon mustard

1 garlic clove, minced

½ cup water

DIRECTIONS

In a small bowl, whisk together all the ingredients, except the water. Gradually stir in the water until the dressing reaches the desired consistency. Store in an airtight container in the refrigerator for up to 5 days.

Nutrition information per serving: *244 calories, 23.2 g fat, 3.3 g saturated fat, 5.3 g protein, 7.7 g carbohydrate, 2.9 g fiber, 518 mg sodium*

Whipped Feta Dip

Serves: 8 / Time: 5 minutes

INGREDIENTS

8 ounces goat feta cheese

¼ cup full-fat organic Greek yogurt

1 teaspoon minced garlic

½ teaspoon sea salt

¼ cup extra virgin olive oil

DIRECTIONS

Crumble the feta into a food processor or a high-speed blender.

Add the Greek yogurt, garlic, and salt. Pulse several times until the feta is fully broken up, scraping down the sides as needed.

Turn the blender on medium speed and slowly add in the olive oil. Turn off, scrape the sides, and blend again.

When the dip reaches the desired consistency, transfer it to a bowl. Top with a bit more olive oil, if desired.

Store in an airtight container in the refrigerator for up to a week.

Nutrition information per serving: *121 calories, 10.6 g fat, 3.4 g saturated fat, 5.6 g protein, 0.4 g carbohydrate, 0 g fiber, 550 mg sodium*

Chili Cheese Dip

Serves: 4 / Time: 20 minutes

INGREDIENTS

4 ounces goat cheese (chèvre)

1 cup Buffalo Chili (page 123), heated up

1 cup crumbled feta cheese

DIRECTIONS

Preheat the oven to 400°F.

Crumble the goat cheese in a small baking dish.

Spread the hot chili on top.

Sprinkle the crumbled feta cheese on top of the chili and bake for 8 to 10 minutes. Store in an airtight container in the refrigerator for up to 3 days.

Nutrition information per serving: *356 calories, 23.3 g fat, 13.2 g saturated fat, 22.9 g protein, 15.8 g carbohydrate, 4.7 g fiber, 1,287 mg sodium*

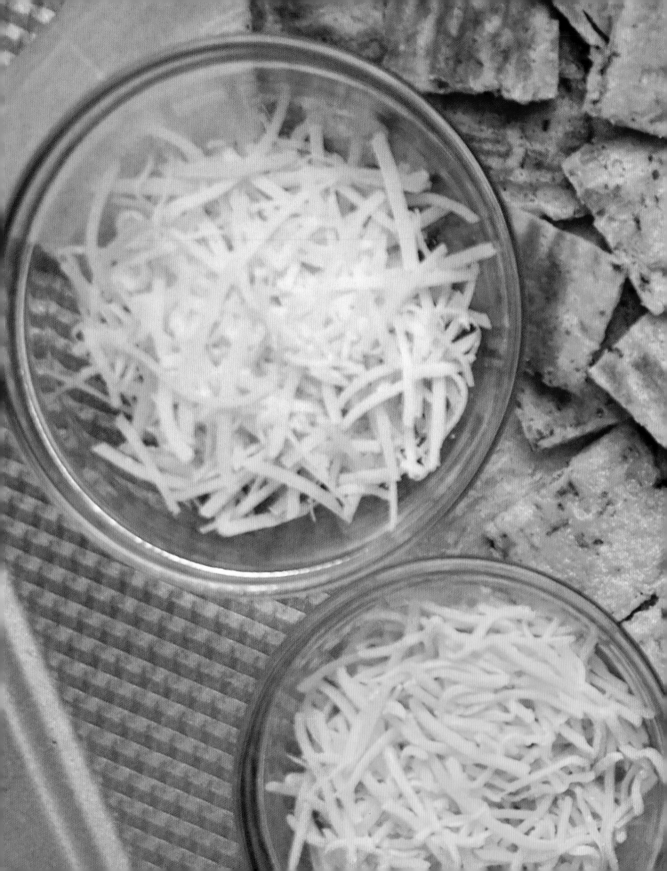

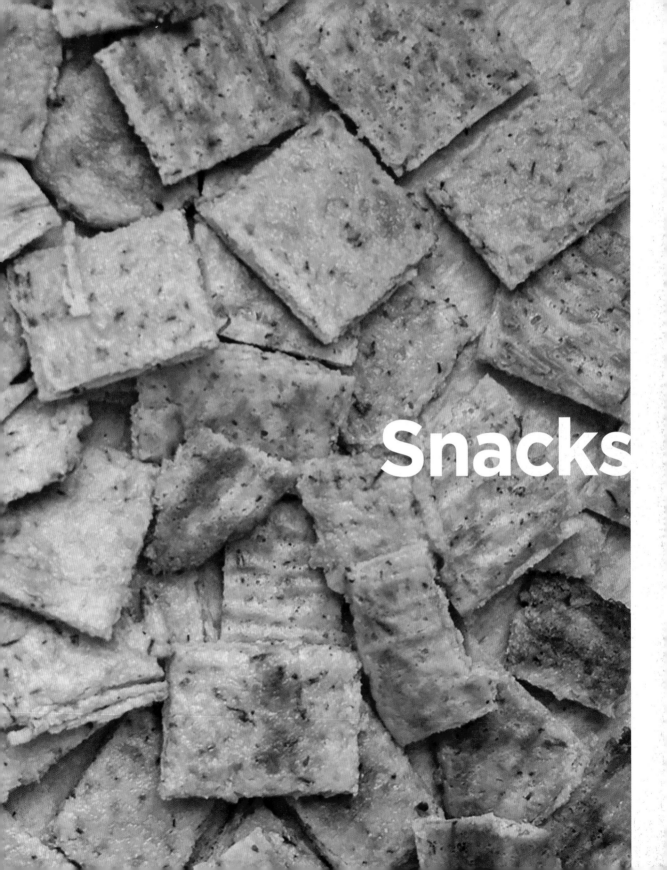

Snacks

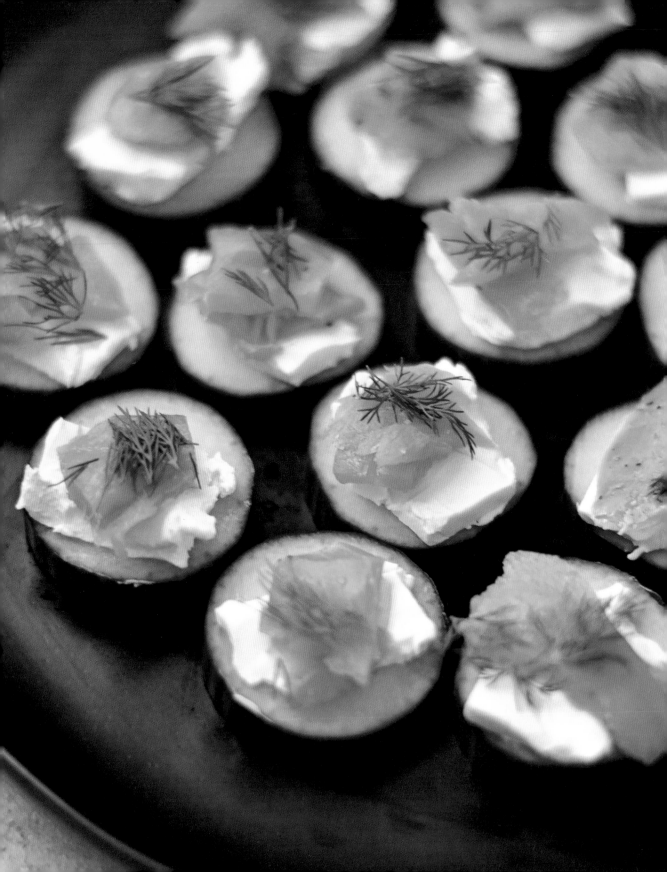

Cucumber
Smoked Salmon Bites

Serves: 4 / Time: 10 minutes

INGREDIENTS

1 English or hothouse
cucumber

2 ounces cream cheese

4 ounces smoked
wild-caught salmon,
skin removed

Fresh dill, to taste
(optional)

DIRECTIONS

Cut the cucumber into ¼-inch-thick slices.

Spread some cream cheese onto each slice. (Tip: This is easier
to do if you first pat the cucumbers dry with a paper towel.)

Cut the smoked salmon into bite-size pieces, roughly the
size of the cucumber slices. Top the cream cheese with
the smoked salmon.

Top with the fresh dill, if using.

Store in the refrigerator in an airtight container for 3 to
4 days.

MAKE IT DAIRY FREE

Use a nut-based or dairy-free cream cheese.

Nutrition information per serving: *103 calories, 7.5 g fat,
3.7 g saturated fat, 8.1 g protein, 0.9 g carbohydrate, 0.3 g fiber,
243 mg sodium*

Jalapeño Poppers

Serves: 6 / Time: 25 minutes

INGREDIENTS

1 cup goat feta cheese

1 cup goat cheese (chèvre)

½ teaspoon cumin

½ teaspoon chili powder

½ teaspoon smoked paprika

½ teaspoon dried oregano

Sea salt and freshly ground black pepper, to taste

12 jalapeño peppers, halved lengthwise, stems and seeds removed

1 (12-ounce) package turkey bacon

DIRECTIONS

Preheat the oven to 350°F. Line a baking sheet with parchment paper.

Put the feta and goat cheeses and all the seasonings into a medium bowl, and mix until well combined.

Fill each jalapeño with the cheese mixture.

Wrap each jalapeño with a slice of turkey bacon and place on the baking sheet.

Bake for 20 minutes, or until the bacon is cooked and crispy, and serve. Store in an airtight container in the refrigerator for up to 3 days.

Nutrition information per serving: *219 calories, 13.1 g fat, 6.7 g saturated fat, 20 g protein, 2.9 g carbohydrate, 1.4 g fiber, 1,489 mg sodium*

Kale Chips

Serves: 4 / Time: 25 minutes

INGREDIENTS

1 bunch kale, stemmed and chopped into 2-inch pieces

2 tablespoons coconut oil, melted and cooled slightly

1 tablespoon lemon juice

¼ teaspoon sea salt

DIRECTIONS

Preheat the oven to 350°F. Line a baking sheet with parchment paper.

Place all the ingredients in a large bowl and, with your hands, massage the oil, lemon juice, and salt into the kale.

Spread the kale on the baking sheet and bake for 12 minutes. Store at room temperature in a sealed plastic bag.

Nutrition information per serving: *101 calories, 6.8 g fat, 5.9 g saturated fat, 2.6 g protein, 9 g carbohydrate, 1.3 g fiber, 155 mg sodium*

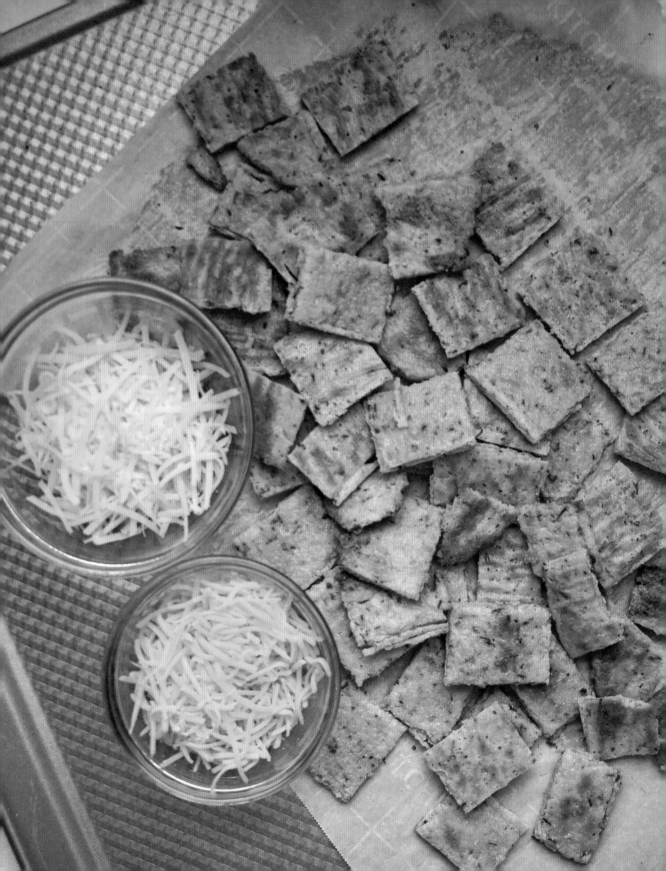

Keto Cheese Crackers

Serves: 8 (5 small crackers per serving) / Time: 24 minutes

INGREDIENTS

1 cup freshly grated Parmesan cheese

1 cup shredded cheddar cheese

2 ounces organic cream cheese

1 cup almond flour

1 large egg

1 teaspoon sea salt

1 tablespoon herbes de Provence

DIRECTIONS

Preheat the oven to 425°F.

In a small pot over medium-low heat, mix together the Parmesan, cheddar, cream cheese, and almond flour. Stir constantly until the cheeses have melted and formed a ball of dough, about 5 minutes.

Remove from the heat and transfer to a mixing bowl. Let cool for 5 minutes.

Mix in the egg, salt, and herbes de Provence.

Place the dough between two large pieces of parchment paper. Using a rolling pin, roll out the dough, about ¼ inch thick or less, into a large rectangle that will fit on your baking sheet. (The thicker the cracker, the longer they will take to bake.)

Carefully remove the top layer of parchment paper and transfer the dough to the baking sheet. Using a pizza cutter or a long, sharp knife, cut the dough into cracker-size squares. Bake for 10 minutes.

Carefully remove the baking sheet from the oven and flip the crackers over. Bake for 3 to 4 minutes, or until both sides have browned nicely and the crackers are crisp.

Let the crackers cool. Store in an airtight container for 3 to 4 days.

Nutrition information per serving: *155 calories, 12.5 g fat, 6.8 g saturated fat, 10 g protein, 1.7 g carbohydrate, 0.4 g fiber, 480 mg sodium*

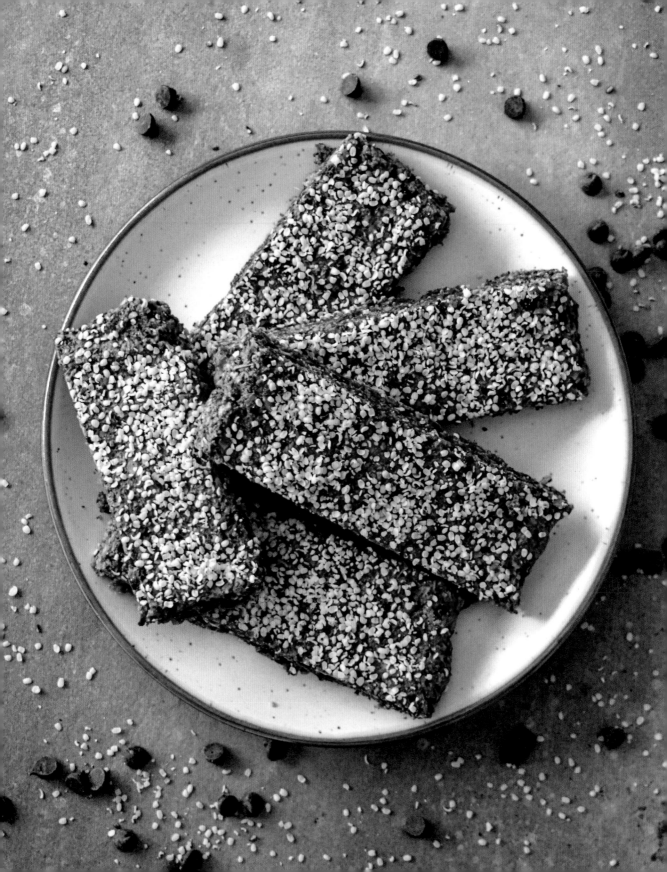

Keto Cookie Dough Bars

Serves: 6 / Time: 30 minutes

INGREDIENTS

⅔ cup cashew or almond butter

½ cup unsweetened chocolate chips

2 scoops vanilla bone broth protein

3 tablespoons coconut cream

1 large egg

DIRECTIONS

Preheat the oven to 325°F. Line a baking sheet with parchment paper.

Put all the ingredients in a food processor and blend well. Stop, scrape down the sides, and blend again.

On a baking sheet, use a rolling pin to shape the dough into a rectangle about ¼ inch thick.

Bake for 20 minutes.

Remove and let cool completely. Cut into six bars. Store in the refrigerator.

MAKE IT VEGAN

Omit the bone broth protein and the egg. Add ½ teaspoon vanilla extract. Bake at 250°F.

Nutrition information per serving: *281 calories, 20.6 g fat, 9.9 g saturated fat, 12.8 g protein, 11.5 g carbohydrate, 3.3 g fiber, 71 mg sodium*

Keto Deviled Eggs

Serves: 6 / Time: 18 minutes

INGREDIENTS

12 large eggs

¼ cup avocado oil mayonnaise

1 tablespoon Dijon mustard

1 teaspoon apple cider vinegar

1 teaspoon dill pickle juice

1 teaspoon sea salt

½ teaspoon freshly ground black pepper

Paprika, to taste

DIRECTIONS

In a large pot, place the eggs in water to cover and bring to a boil over medium-high heat. Cover the pot and turn off the heat. Let the eggs sit for 8 minutes.

Remove the eggs with a slotted spoon and cool them in a large bowl of ice water.

When the eggs are cool, remove the shells and slice in half lengthwise. Carefully remove the yolks and put them in a medium mixing bowl.

Add the remaining ingredients, except the paprika, to the yolks and whisk together until blended.

Spoon or pipe the yolk mixture into each egg half.

Sprinkle with the paprika and enjoy. Store in the refrigerator.

Nutrition information per serving: *98 calories, 8.1 g fat, 1.9 g saturated fat, 5.6 g protein, 0.5 g carbohydrate, 0.1 g fiber, 270 mg sodium*

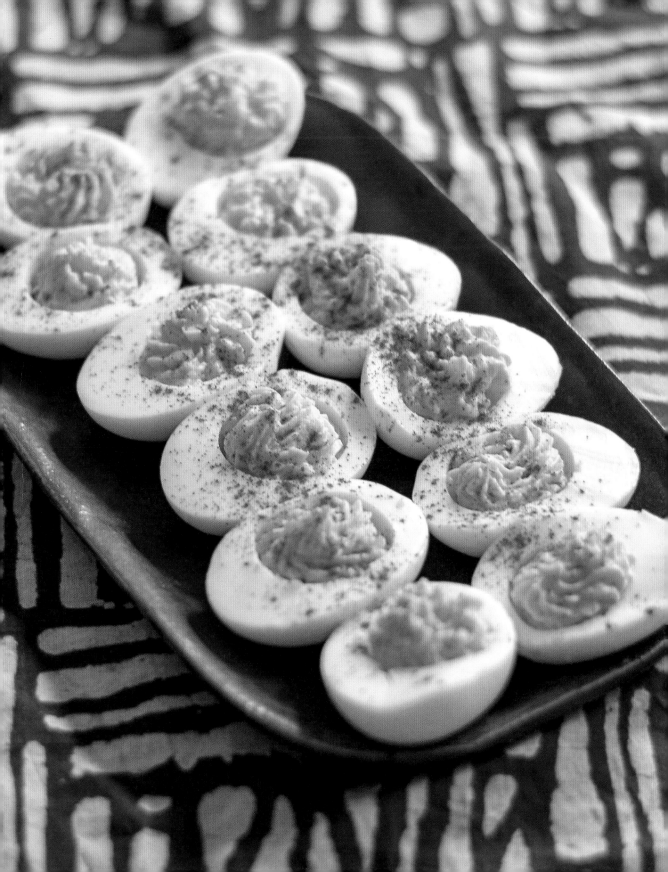

Keto Bread

Serves: 10 / Time: 40 minutes

INGREDIENTS

¼ teaspoon cream of tartar

6 large egg whites

1½ cups almond flour

4 tablespoons butter, melted

¾ teaspoon baking soda

3 teaspoons apple cider vinegar

2 tablespoons coconut flour

DIRECTIONS

Preheat the oven to 375°F. Grease an 8 x 4-inch loaf pan.

In a medium bowl, combine the cream of tartar and the egg whites. Beat the egg whites with an electric mixer until they form soft peaks.

Put the almond flour, butter, baking soda, apple cider vinegar, and coconut flour in a food processor, and blend until well combined.

Remove the mixture to a large bowl and gently fold in the egg whites.

Pour the batter into the loaf pan and bake for 30 minutes.

Remove from the oven and let cool for 10 minutes. Store in the refrigerator.

Nutrition information per serving: *44 calories, 3.5 g fat, 1.6 g saturated fat, 1.8 g protein, 1.6 g carbohydrate, 0.8 g fiber, 73 mg sodium*

Keto Fat Bombs

Serves: 12 / Time: 1 hour

INGREDIENTS

1 stick (½ cup) butter

½ cup crunchy
almond butter

1 teaspoon vanilla extract

½ teaspoon cinnamon

DIRECTIONS

Line a 12-cup muffin pan with paper liners.

In a small saucepan over medium-low heat, melt the butter and almond butter. Remove from the heat.

Add the vanilla and cinnamon, stirring until well combined.

Fill the muffin cups equally with the mixture.

Freeze for 30 minutes to 1 hour. Store in refrigerator.

Nutrition information per serving: *199 calories, 19 g fat, 5.5 g saturated fat, 5.4 g protein, 4.1 g carbohydrate, 2.1 g fiber, 54 mg sodium*

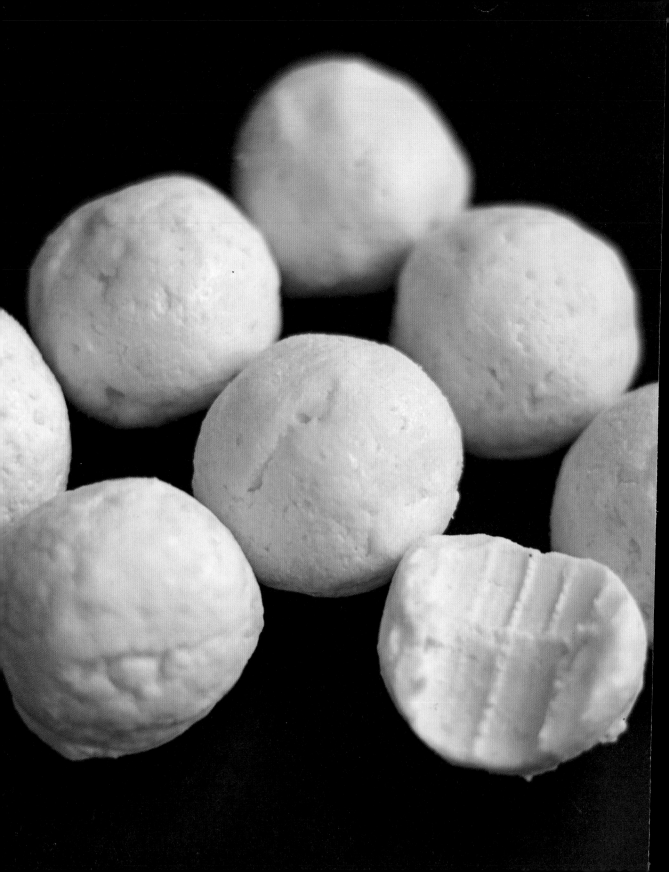

Lemon Coconut Cheesecake Fat Bombs

Serves: 12 / Chill Time: 1 hour, 10 minutes

INGREDIENTS

4 ounces full-fat cream cheese, softened

¼ cup coconut butter

3 tablespoons coconut flour

2 tablespoons monk fruit powdered sweetener

Zest of 1 lemon

Juice of ½ lemon

½ teaspoon vanilla extract

DIRECTIONS

Line a baking sheet with parchment paper.

In a small bowl, beat the cream cheese and coconut butter together with a handheld or stand mixer.

Add the remaining ingredients and beat on medium speed until well combined.

Place the dough in the refrigerator to chill for 30 minutes.

Roll the dough into balls using 2 tablespoons of dough. Set the balls on the baking sheet. Repeat until all the dough is used.

Place the baking sheet in the freezer for 30 minutes, or until hard. Store in an airtight container in the freezer or in the refrigerator.

Nutrition information per serving: *131 calories, 11.5 g fat, 3.5 g saturated fat, 5.1 g protein, 6.8 g carbohydrate, 1.5 g fiber, 52 mg sodium*

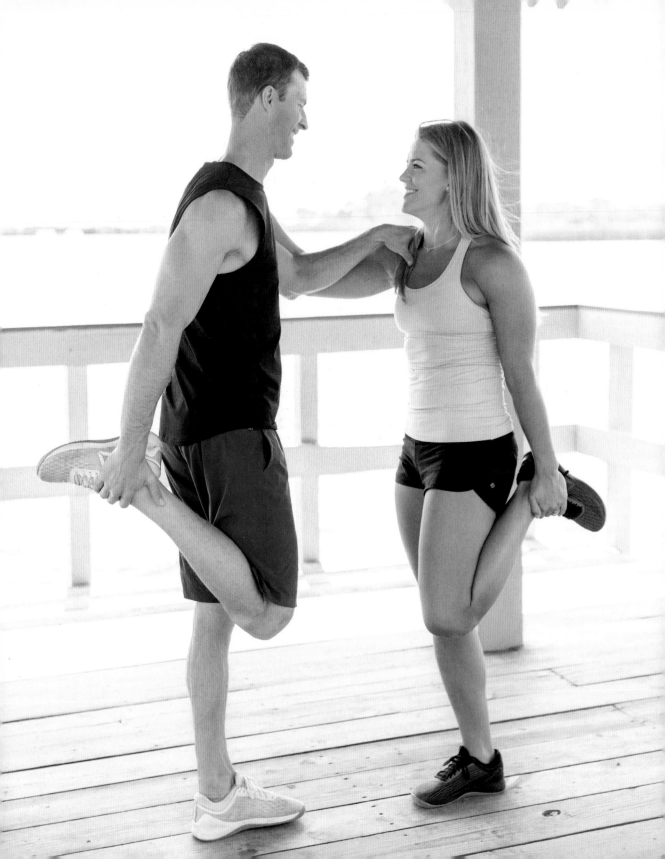

Roasted Mixed Nuts

Serves: 4 / Time: 20 minutes

INGREDIENTS

1 cup raw pecans

1 cup raw cashews

1 cup raw almonds

1 cup raw walnuts

3 tablespoons coconut oil, melted

1 tablespoon sea salt

1 teaspoon cayenne pepper (optional)

DIRECTIONS

Preheat the oven to 350°F. Line a baking sheet with parchment paper.

Toss all the ingredients together in a mixing bowl until the nuts are evenly coated with oil.

Spread the nuts out on the baking sheet and bake for 14 to 16 minutes, until lightly browned and fragrant. Remove and let cool. Store in a glass container at room temperature.

Nutrition information per serving: *674 calories, 62.2 g fat, 15.7 g saturated fat, 18.6 g protein, 20.6 g carbohydrate, 7 g fiber, 1,411 mg sodium*

Spicy Roasted Pumpkin Seeds

Serves: 8 / Time: 10 minutes

INGREDIENTS

4 tablespoons coconut oil

2 cups raw pumpkin seeds

4 teaspoons Tabasco sauce

½ teaspoon cayenne pepper

DIRECTIONS

Line a baking sheet with parchment paper.

Heat the oil in a large pan over medium heat.

Add the pumpkin seeds and sauté for 2 to 3 minutes, or until they start to pop and turn golden brown.

Add the Tabasco and cayenne, toss, and continue to cook for 1 minute.

Transfer to the baking sheet, carefully spread the seeds out in a single layer, and let cool before serving. Store in a glass container at room temperature.

Nutrition information per serving: *246 calories, 22.7 g fat, 8.9 g saturated fat, 8.5 g protein, 6.2 g carbohydrate, 1.4 g fiber, 21 mg sodium*

Zucchini Pizza Bites

Serves: 2 / Time: 10 minutes

INGREDIENTS

1 large zucchini

1 tablespoon extra virgin olive oil

¼ cup organic marinara sauce (no sugar added)

2 tablespoons organic shredded mozzarella cheese

2 tablespoons freshly grated Parmesan cheese

DIRECTIONS

Preheat the oven to broil.

Slice the zucchini into ¼-inch-thick slices. Put them on a baking sheet and put it under the broiler for 3 minutes.

Remove the baking sheet and turn the slices over. Brush the tops with the olive oil and put under the broiler for 3 minutes.

Carefully remove the baking sheet and cover the slices evenly with the marinara sauce and cheeses. Put under the broiler for 2 to 3 minutes, or until the cheeses have melted.

Carefully remove the baking sheet from the broiler and let the bites cool to warm before serving.

MAKE IT VEGAN AND DAIRY FREE
Use dairy-free and vegan cheeses.

Nutrition information per serving: *206 calories, 14 g fat, 5.1 g saturated fat, 12.7 g protein, 10.2 g carbohydrate, 2.3 g fiber, 366 mg sodium*

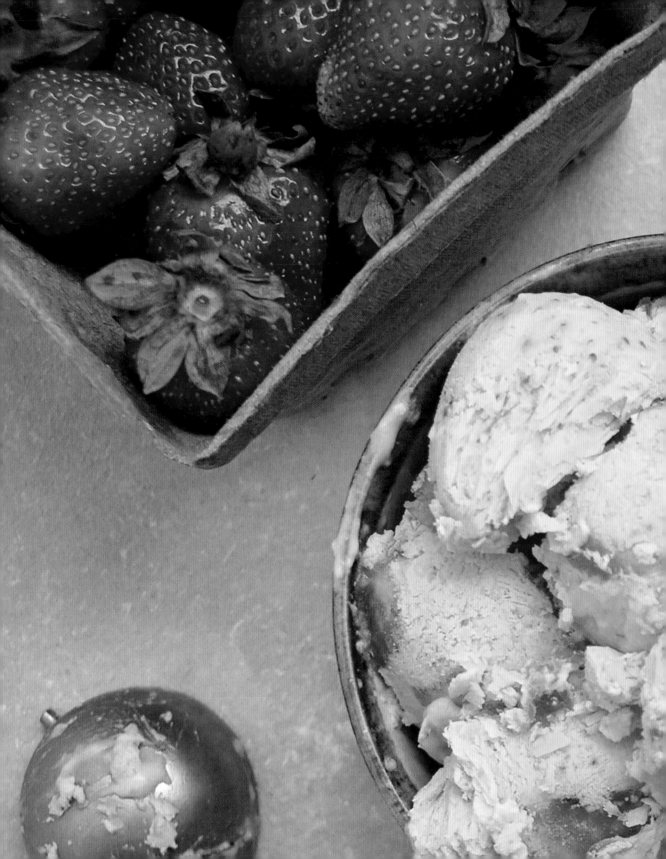

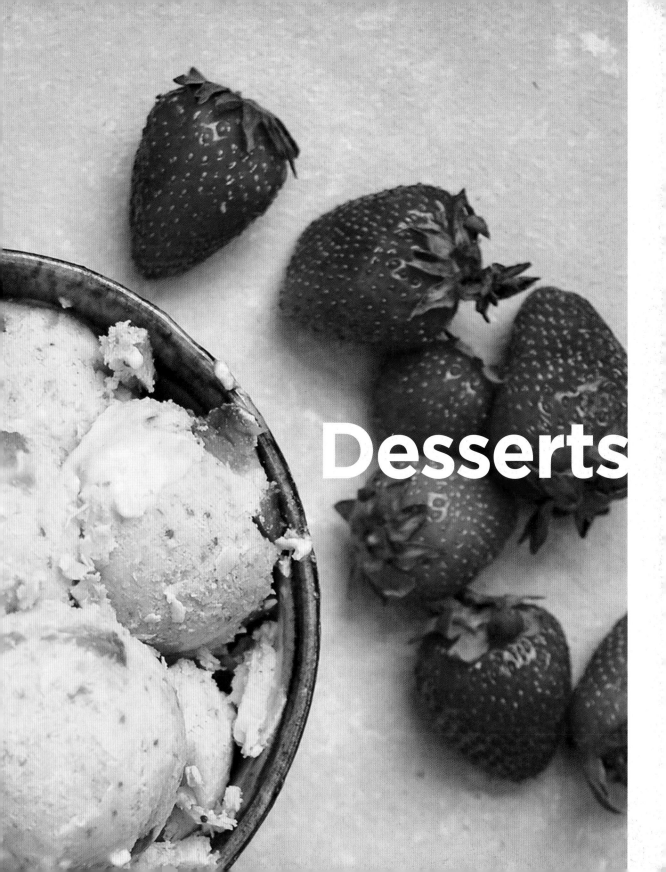

Desserts

Almond Butter Cups

Serves: 12 / Time: 1 hour, 10 minutes

INGREDIENTS

¼ **cup all-natural almond butter**

1 **tablespoon coconut flour**

1 **tablespoon plus 1 teaspoon coconut oil**

¾ **cup stevia-sweetened dark chocolate chips**

2 **teaspoons hemp CBD oil (see Note)**

DIRECTIONS

Line a 12-cup mini muffin pan with paper liners.

In a small bowl, stir together the almond butter and coconut flour. Set aside.

Melt the coconut oil and the dark chocolate chips together, either in the microwave in a microwave-safe bowl in 30-second increments, or in a double boiler.

Stir the CBD oil into the melted chocolate.

Spoon half of the chocolate into the muffin cups and tilt them so a little goes up the sides.

Scoop about ¼ teaspoon of the almond butter mixture into each cup.

Cover with the remaining chocolate. Place in the refrigerator for 1 hour, or until set. Store in refrigerator.

NOTE: If you choose to omit the CBD oil, use 2 teaspoons coconut oil instead.

Nutrition information per serving: *137 calories, 11.3 g fat, 4.9 g saturated fat, 3.2 g protein, 11.2 g carbohydrate, 3.5 g fiber, 22 mg sodium*

Chocolate Muffins

Serves: 12 / Time: 25 minutes

INGREDIENTS

3 large eggs

¼ cup coconut oil, melted

1 full dropper liquid vanilla stevia

1 teaspoon vanilla extract

⅛ teaspoon apple cider vinegar

1 cup almond flour

3 tablespoons xanthan gum

1½ tablespoons ground flax seeds

1 teaspoon baking powder

½ teaspoon cinnamon

½ teaspoon salt

1 cup cacao nibs

3 scoops chocolate bone broth protein

DIRECTIONS

Preheat the oven to 375°F. Line a 12-cup muffin pan with paper liners.

In a large mixing bowl, whisk the eggs until light in color. Add the coconut oil, stevia, vanilla extract, and vinegar. Whisk to combine.

In a medium bowl, combine the dry ingredients together until well blended. Add the dry ingredients to the wet ingredients. Stir to combine thoroughly and let the mixture sit for 2 minutes.

Put the batter into the muffin cups, filling them three-quarters full. Bake for 13 to 15 minutes, or until golden brown. Store in the refrigerator.

Nutrition information per serving: *196 calories, 12.9 g fat, 5.9 g saturated fat, 11 g protein, 21.8 g carbohydrate, 18.1 g fiber, 574 mg sodium*

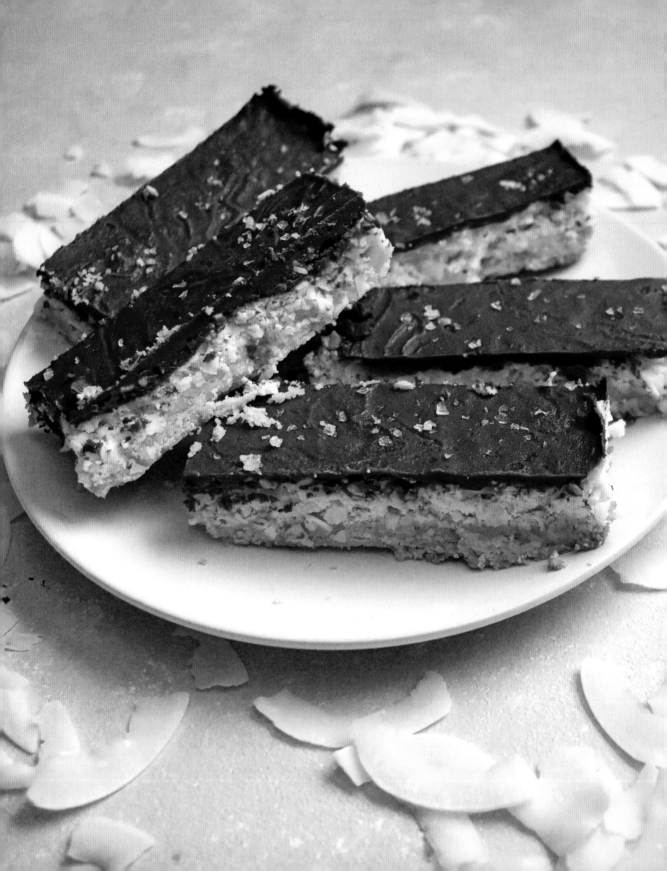

Coconut Chocolate Bars

Serves: 12 / Time: 1 hour, 30 minutes

INGREDIENTS

Crust:

6 tablespoons cultured butter, melted (or ghee)

2 cups almond flour

1½ tablespoons stevia (about 10 packets)

Pinch of salt

Coconut Layer:

2 cups unsweetened coconut flakes

⅔ cup full-fat coconut milk

¼ cup coconut oil, melted

¼ cup monk fruit syrup, maple flavored

¼ teaspoon almond extract

Chocolate Layer:

½ cup coconut oil, melted

¼ cup plus 2 tablespoons monk fruit syrup, maple flavored

½ cup unsweetened cocoa powder

DIRECTIONS

Preheat the oven to 350°F. Line an 8 x 8-inch baking pan with parchment paper.

Combine all the crust ingredients and press into the pan. Bake for 15 minutes. Remove from the oven and let cool.

To make the coconut layer, put all the ingredients in a food processor and pulse until fully combined. Pour on top of the crust layer and place in the refrigerator for 15 minutes.

To make the chocolate layer, warm the coconut oil and syrup in a small saucepan and stir well. Add the cocoa powder and stir until combined. Pour over the coconut layer and return the pan to the refrigerator for 30 minutes to 1 hour, or until set.

Cut and serve cold. Store in the refrigerator.

Nutrition information per serving: *327 calories, 33.4 g fat, 26.5 g saturated fat, 2.3 g protein, 6.2 g carbohydrate, 3.9 g fiber, 80 mg sodium*

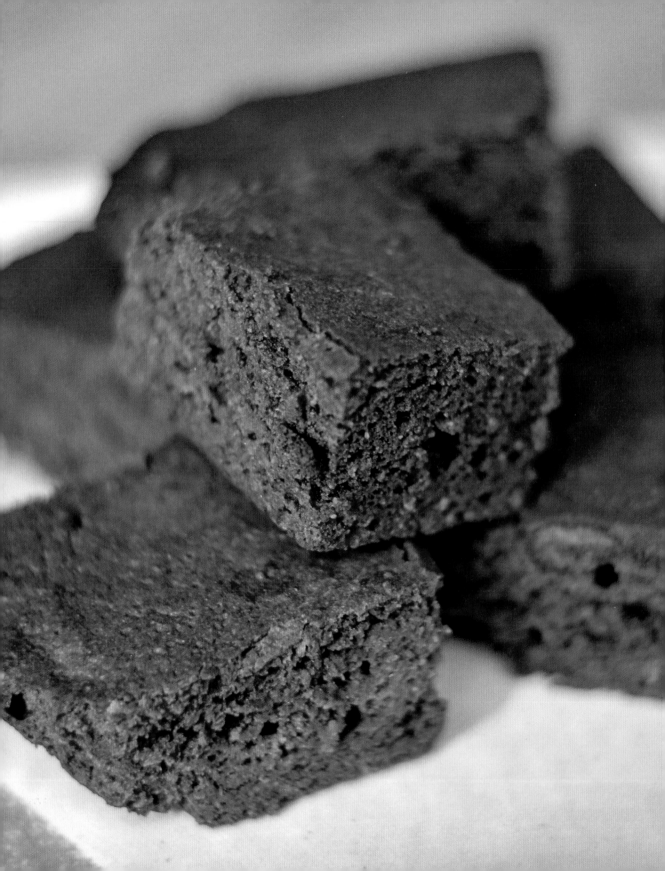

Keto Brownies

Serves: 16 / Time: 50 minutes

INGREDIENTS

½ cup almond flour

¼ cup unsweetened cocoa powder

½ teaspoon sea salt

½ teaspoon baking powder

2 ounces unsweetened dark chocolate

½ cup coconut oil

½ cup monk fruit sweetener

3 large eggs, at room temperature

½ teaspoon vanilla extract

DIRECTIONS

Preheat the oven to 350°F. Line an 8 x 8-inch baking pan with parchment paper.

In a medium bowl, mix together the flour, cocoa powder, salt, and baking powder.

In a double boiler or microwave, melt the dark chocolate and coconut oil together and stir until smooth. (If using the microwave, heat at 30-second intervals, stirring between intervals.)

In a large bowl, beat the sweetener, eggs, and vanilla together vigorously. Add the chocolate mixture and continue to mix.

Fold in the flour mixture and mix until the batter is smooth.

Pour the batter into the baking pan and bake for 20 minutes, or until a toothpick inserted into the center comes out clean. Cut into 16 brownies and serve. Store in the refrigerator.

MAKE IT VEGAN
Replace the eggs with 3 tablespoons flaxseed powder plus ½ cup water.

GIVE IT A COLLAGEN BOOST
Add 2 scoops collagen protein to the flour mixture.

Nutrition information per serving: *139 calories, 13.1 g fat, 9.3 g saturated fat, 3.2 g protein, 10.9 g carbohydrate, 2.6 g fiber, 73 mg sodium*

Coffee Cake

Serves: 9 / Time: 55 minutes

INGREDIENTS

Cake:

2 tablespoons coconut oil, melted

1 large egg

1 teaspoon vanilla extract

1 teaspoon liquid stevia

½ cup coconut milk

1½ cups blanched almond flour

1 teaspoon cinnamon

2 teaspoons baking powder

½ teaspoon sea salt

Topping:

½ cup blanched almond flour

1½ tablespoons coconut oil, melted

5 drops liquid stevia

2 teaspoons cinnamon

DIRECTIONS

Preheat the oven to 350°F. Grease an 8 x 8-inch baking dish or loaf pan.

In a large bowl, combine the coconut oil, egg, vanilla extract, stevia, and coconut milk, and stir until well combined.

In a medium bowl, combine the almond flour, cinnamon, baking powder, and salt.

Add the dry ingredients to the wet ingredients and stir until smooth.

Pour the batter into the greased baking dish.

In a small bowl, mix the topping ingredients together and crumble over the cake.

Bake for 45 to 50 minutes. Remove from the oven, test doneness with a toothpick, let cool, and remove from the baking dish. Serve warm. Store in the refrigerator.

Nutrition information per serving: *130 calories, 12.3 g fat, 8.5 g saturated fat, 2.4 g protein, 2.9 g carbohydrate, 1.4 g fiber, 117 mg sodium*

Keto Cheesecake

Serves: 12 / Time: 3 hours, 30 minutes

INGREDIENTS

Crust:

1½ cups almond flour

1 packet stevia

5 tablespoons butter, melted

1 teaspoon pure vanilla extract

Filling:

24 ounces cream cheese, softened

1 tablespoon stevia (about 5 packets)

½ cup coconut cream

2 large eggs

1 teaspoon lemon zest

Blueberry topping (optional):

1 cup blueberries

5 drops liquid stevia

DIRECTIONS

Preheat the oven to 350°F.

In a small bowl, mix together the crust ingredients. Press into the bottom of a 9-inch springform pan and bake for 10 minutes. Remove and let cool.

Reduce the oven temperature to 300°F.

To make the filling, in a medium bowl, mix together the cream cheese and stevia. Slowly add the coconut cream and mix until fully incorporated. Scrape down the sides of the bowl.

Add the eggs one at a time, whisking during each addition. Add the lemon zest and stir in.

Pour the cream cheese mixture into the pan and place in the oven.

Bake for 1 hour. Remove from the oven and check for doneness by gently shaking the cheesecake, making sure only the center circle jiggles. Let the cheesecake cool completely. Chill in the refrigerator for 3 hours (or overnight) before removing it from the pan.

In a small saucepan over low heat, warm the blueberries and stevia together, and slightly mash the blueberries with a fork. Serve on top of the cheesecake. Store in an airtight container in the refrigerator for up to 3 days.

Nutrition information per serving: *345 calories, 34.9 g fat, 21.4 g saturated fat, 6.3 g protein, 3.1 g carbohydrate, 0.6 g fiber, 230 mg sodium*

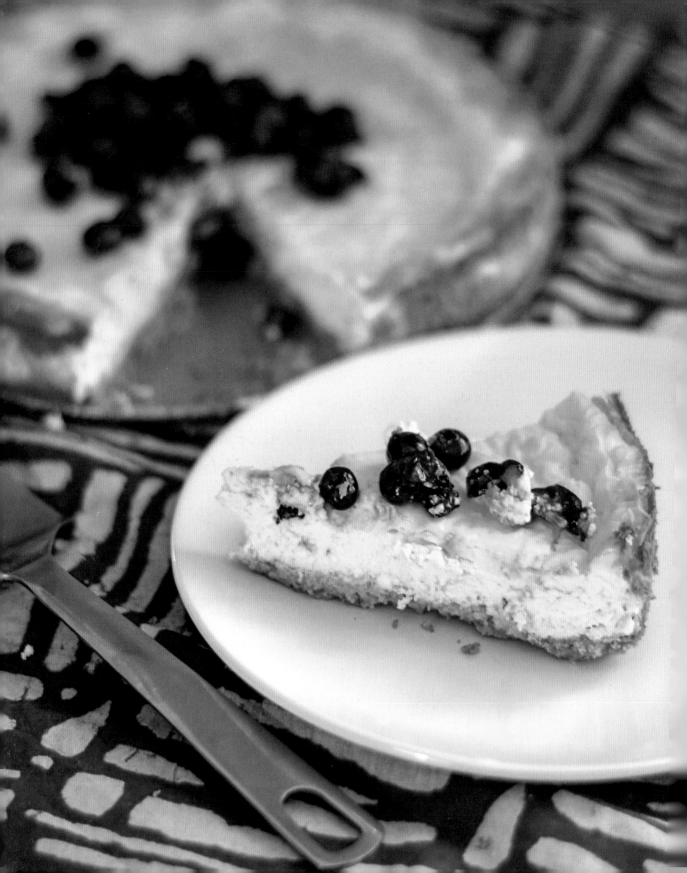

Vegan Keto Cheesecake

Serves: 12 / Time: 1 hour, 25 minutes

INGREDIENTS

Crust:

1½ cups almond flour

1 packet stevia

5 tablespoons coconut oil, melted

1 teaspoon pure vanilla extract

Filling:

16 ounces cashew vegan cream cheese

1 cup unsweetened coconut yogurt

1 teaspoon lemon zest

1 teaspoon lemon juice

1 tablespoon stevia (about 5 packets)

2 tablespoons coconut oil, melted

DIRECTIONS

Preheat the oven to 350°F.

In a small bowl, mix together the crust ingredients. Press into the bottom of a 9-inch springform pan and bake for 10 minutes. Remove and let cool.

In a medium bowl, whisk together all the filling ingredients until incorporated and creamy. Pour on top of the baked crust and freeze for about 1 hour. Once firm, it is ready to enjoy. Store in an airtight container in the refrigerator for up to 3 days.

Nutrition information per serving: *328 calories, 29 g fat, 20.2 g saturated fat, 8 g protein, 11 g carbohydrate, 0.5 g fiber, 166 mg sodium*

Keto Chocolate Chip Cookies

Serves: 24 / Time: 22 minutes

INGREDIENTS

2 cups almond flour

1 scoop collagen protein

½ teaspoon baking powder

¼ teaspoon sea salt

½ cup coconut oil, melted

½ cup monk fruit sweetener

1 teaspoon pure
vanilla extract

2 large eggs

½ cup unsweetened
chocolate chips

DIRECTIONS

Preheat the oven to 350°F. Line a baking sheet with parchment paper.

In a large bowl, mix together the almond flour, collagen protein, baking powder, and sea salt. Set aside.

In a small bowl, mix together the coconut oil, monk fruit sweetener, vanilla, and eggs.

Incorporate the coconut oil mixture into the flour mixture until a thick dough forms. Stir in the chocolate chips.

Scoop and roll the dough into 24 balls and gently flatten with the back of a spoon or your fingertips. Place them 2 inches apart on the prepared baking sheet.

Bake for 10 to 12 minutes. Remove from the sheet and allow to cool on a wire rack. Store in the refrigerator.

Nutrition information per serving: *54 calories, 4.2 g fat, 1.9 g saturated fat, 2.0 g protein, 5.9 g carbohydrate, 0.9 g fiber, 26 mg sodium*

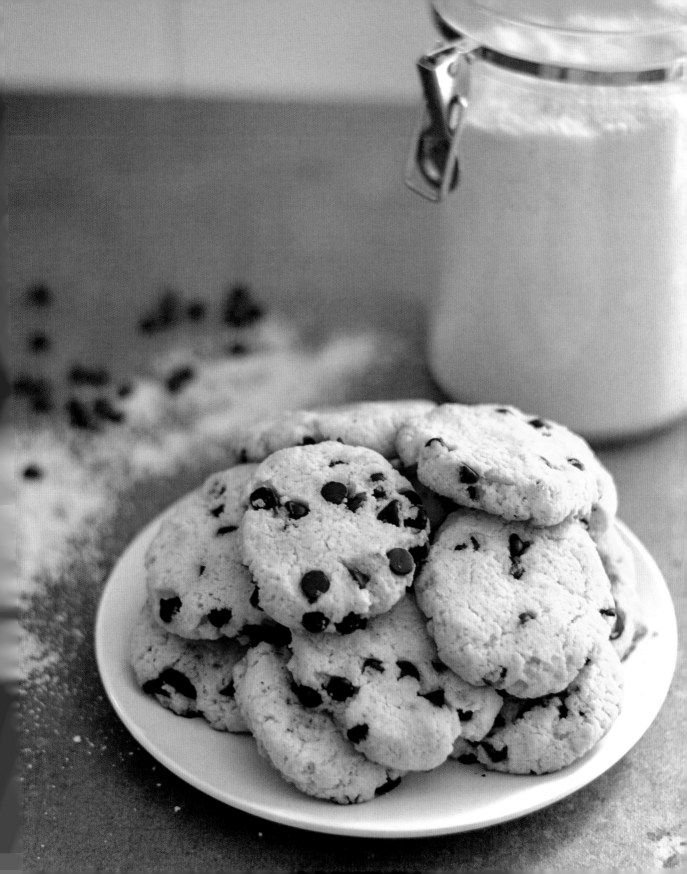

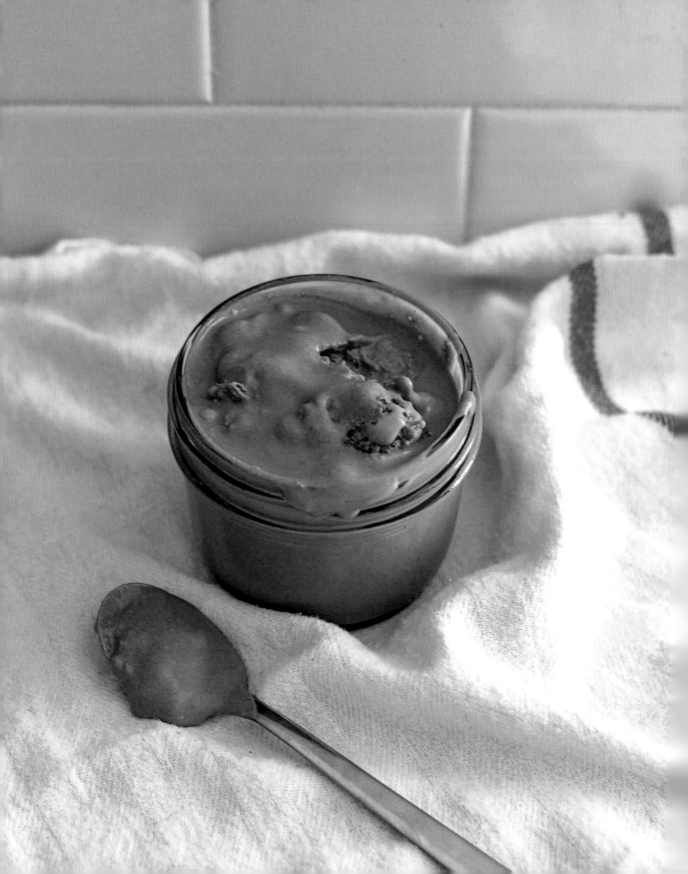

Keto Chocolate Frosty

Serves: 1 / Time: 35 minutes

INGREDIENTS

1 cup full fat coconut milk

2 tablespoons cocoa powder

1 tablespoon almond butter

1 teaspoon vanilla extract

1 tablespoon stevia (about 5 packets)

DIRECTIONS

In a medium bowl, whisk together all the ingredients with an electric hand mixer, stand mixer, or a hand-whisk for 30 seconds, or until the ingredients are fully incorporated, thick, and creamy.

Freeze for 30 minutes. Whisk again for smoothness and enjoy.

GIVE IT A COLLAGEN BOOST

Add 1 scoop of keto collagen powder.

Nutrition information per serving: *579 calories, 58.6 g fat, 44.3 g saturated fat, 9.9 g protein, 15.8 g carbohydrate, 4.8 g fiber, 33 mg sodium*

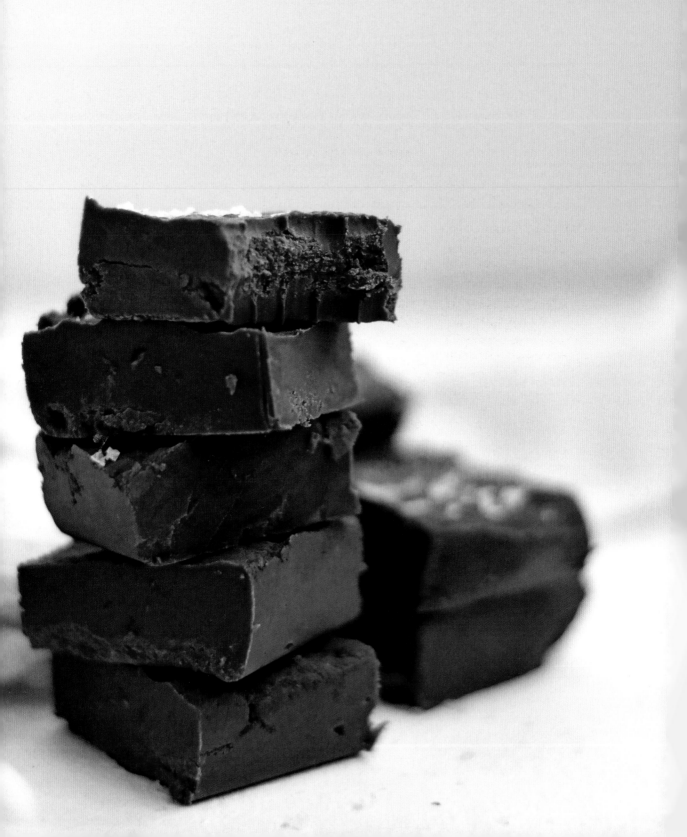

Keto Fudge

Serves: 10 / Time: 3 hours

INGREDIENTS

1 cup full-fat coconut cream

¼ cup powdered monk fruit sweetener

2 teaspoons vanilla extract

2 tablespoons butter, room temperature

1 cup stevia-sweetened dark chocolate chips

DIRECTIONS

Line a loaf pan with parchment paper.

In a small saucepan over medium heat, bring the coconut cream, monk fruit sweetener, and vanilla to a simmer, stirring often. Simmer for 20 minutes, or until it has reduced by nearly half and has the consistency of condensed milk.

Reduce the heat to low and stir in the butter until it has melted.

Stir in the dark chocolate chips until they have melted.

Remove from the heat and pour into the prepared loaf pan. Place in the refrigerator for at least 2 hours, or until the fudge has set. Turn upside down on a wooden cutting board and pop out. Use a sharp, heavy knife to carefully cut 1-inch square pieces. Store in the refrigerator.

Nutrition information per serving: *166 calories, 14.4 g fat, 10.5 g saturated fat, 2.2 g protein, 17.4 g carbohydrate, 3.7 g fiber, 20 mg sodium*

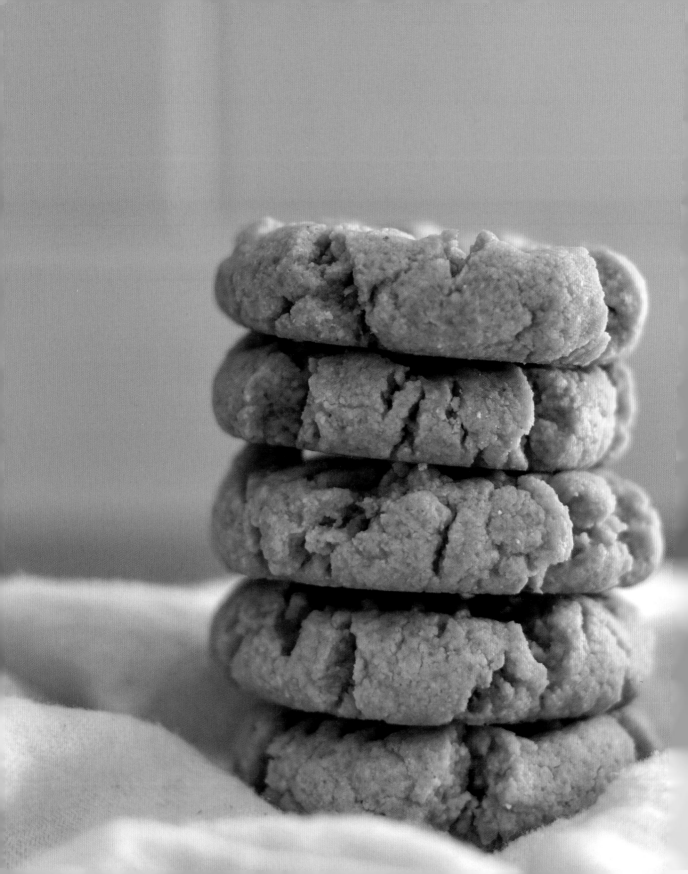

Keto Peanut Butter Cookies

Serves: 12 / Time: 22 minutes

INGREDIENTS

1 cup all-natural peanut butter

⅓ cup monk fruit sweetener

⅔ cup almond flour

1 large egg

1 scoop keto collagen powder

¼ teaspoon sea salt

DIRECTIONS

Preheat the oven to 350°F. Line a baking sheet with parchment paper.

In a medium bowl, combine all the ingredients and mix well.

Using 2 tablespoons of dough, form equal-size balls and place them on the prepared baking sheet, about 2 inches apart. Using a fork, press the balls down in a crosshatch pattern.

Bake for 12 minutes. Remove from the oven and allow to cool on a wire rack. Store in the refrigerator.

MAKE IT VEGAN

Replace the egg with 1 tablespoon flaxseed powder plus 3 tablespoons water. Omit the keto collagen powder, and add ¼ teaspoon vanilla extract.

Nutrition information per serving: *44 calories, 2.4 g fat, 0.6 g saturated fat, 2.4 g protein, 9.3 g carbohydrate, 0.5 g fiber, 50 mg sodium*

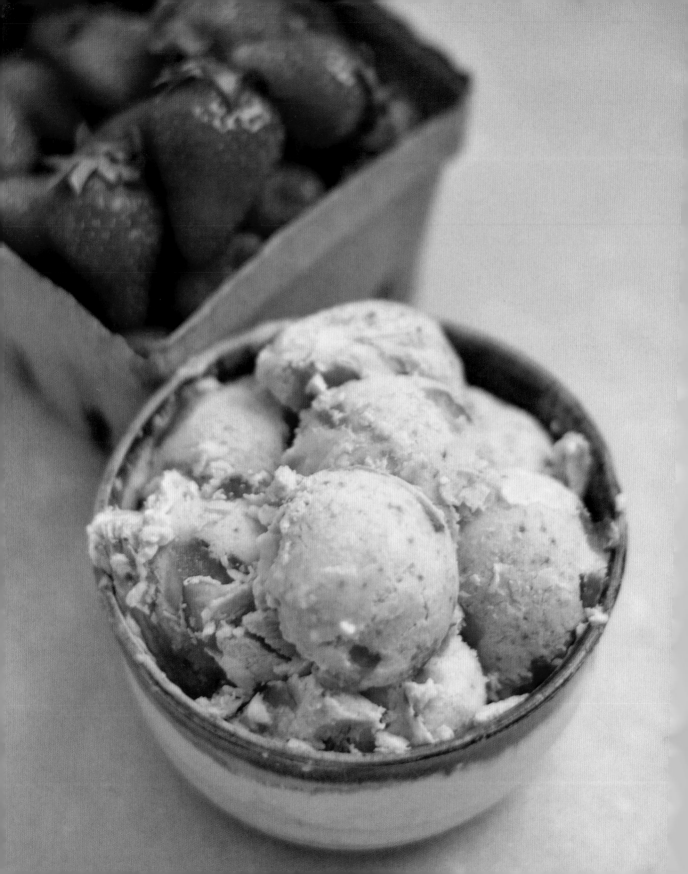

Keto Strawberry Ice Cream

Serves: 4 / Time: 3 to 4 hours

INGREDIENTS

2 cups full-fat coconut milk

½ cup monk fruit sweetener

2 tablespoons MCT oil

1 teaspoon vanilla extract

1 heaping cup strawberries,
divided

DIRECTIONS

Put the coconut milk, monk fruit sweetener, MCT oil, vanilla extract, and half of the strawberries in a high-speed blender and blend well.

Dice the other half of the strawberries and stir into the ice cream mixture.

Pour into a freezerproof glass container and place in the freezer for 3 to 4 hours, or until set.

Remove from the freezer and let the ice cream sit at room temperature for about 10 minutes before serving. Scoop and enjoy.

Nutrition information per serving: *341 calories, 35.7 g fat, 32.4 g saturated fat, 3 g protein, 13.6 g carbohydrate, 3.4 g fiber, 18 mg sodium*

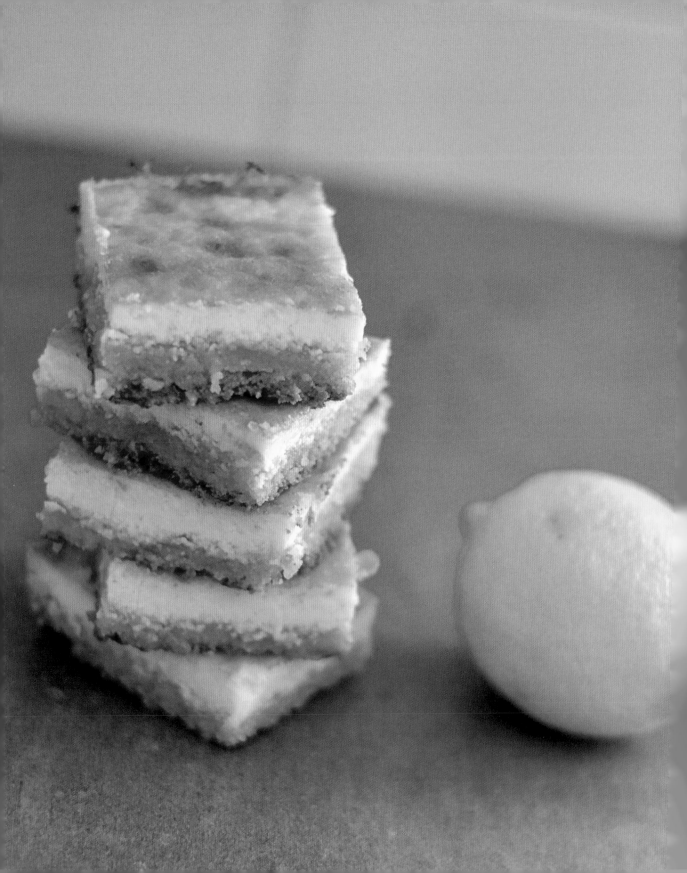

Lemon Bars

Serves: 16 / Time: 2 hours, 50 minutes

INGREDIENTS

Crust:

6 tablespoons ghee or grass-fed butter, softened

2 cups almond flour

2 tablespoons stevia (about 10 packets)

1 tablespoon lemon zest

Filling:

½ cup ghee or grass-fed butter, melted

2 scoops collagen protein

3 large eggs

½ cup lemon juice

2 tablespoons stevia (about 10 packets)

4 drops liquid stevia

2 tablespoons lemon zest

Pinch of sea salt

DIRECTIONS

Preheat the oven to 350°F. Line an 8 x 8-inch baking pan with parchment paper.

In a medium bowl, combine all the ingredients for the crust and press into the bottom of the pan. Bake for 10 minutes.

To make the filling, in a medium bowl, whisk together the melted ghee and collagen protein.

Add the remaining filling ingredients to the butter mixture. Pour over the baked crust. Put the pan in the oven.

Bake for 20 minutes. Remove and let cool, then place in the refrigerator for at least 2 hours, or until fully set. Cut into 16 servings and store in the refrigerator.

Nutrition information per serving: *121 calories, 11.2 g fat, 5.8 g saturated fat, 3.1 g protein, 2.4 g carbohydrate, 0.5 g fiber, 31 mg sodium*

Toasted
Coconut Macaroons

Serves: 12 / Time: 45 minutes

INGREDIENTS

2 cups unsweetened shredded coconut

2 egg whites

¼ cup monk fruit sweetener

½ teaspoon baking powder

½ teaspoon pure vanilla or almond extract

Pinch of sea salt

¼ cup 80% (or higher) dark chocolate, melted (optional)

DIRECTIONS

Preheat the oven to 350°F. Line a baking pan with parchment paper.

Place the shredded coconut in the baking pan and toast for 5 minutes.

Let cool. Reduce the oven to 325°F.

In a medium bowl, beat the egg whites with a handheld mixer until they form soft peaks. While whisking gently, slowly add the monk fruit sweetener, baking powder, vanilla, and sea salt.

Gently fold in the toasted coconut until fully incorporated.

With your hands, form 10 to 12 equal-size balls and place them on the prepared baking sheet.

Bake for 10 minutes. Reduce the heat to 300°F and bake for 20 minutes.

Remove and let cool. When cooled, dip the bottoms into the melted chocolate, if desired, and return to the parchment paper. When the chocolate has hardened, serve and enjoy. Store in the refrigerator.

Nutrition information per serving: *254 calories, 21.9 g fat, 19.1 g saturated fat, 3.4 g protein, 13.4 g carbohydrate, 5.3 g fiber, 39 mg sodium*

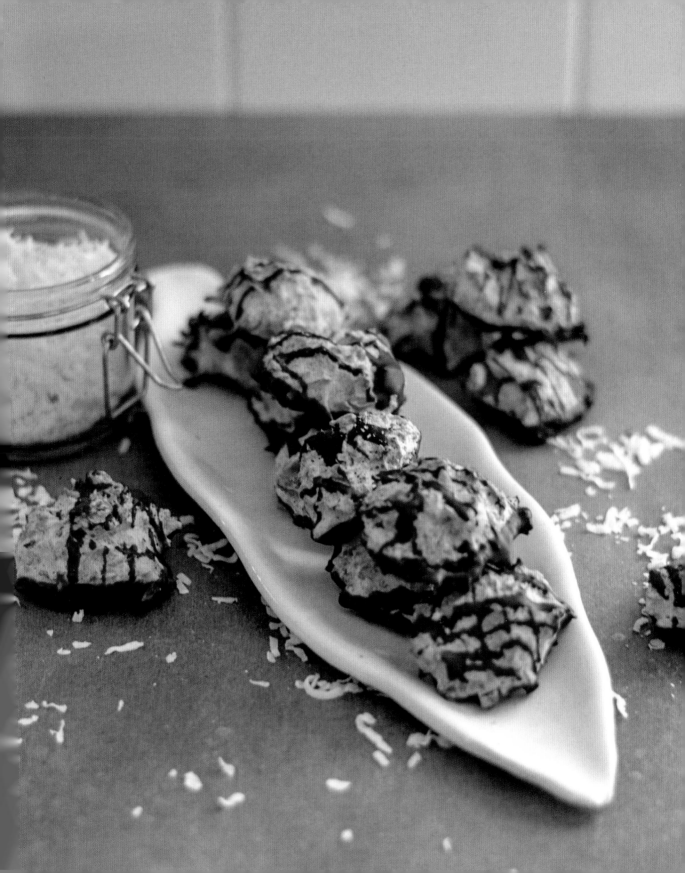

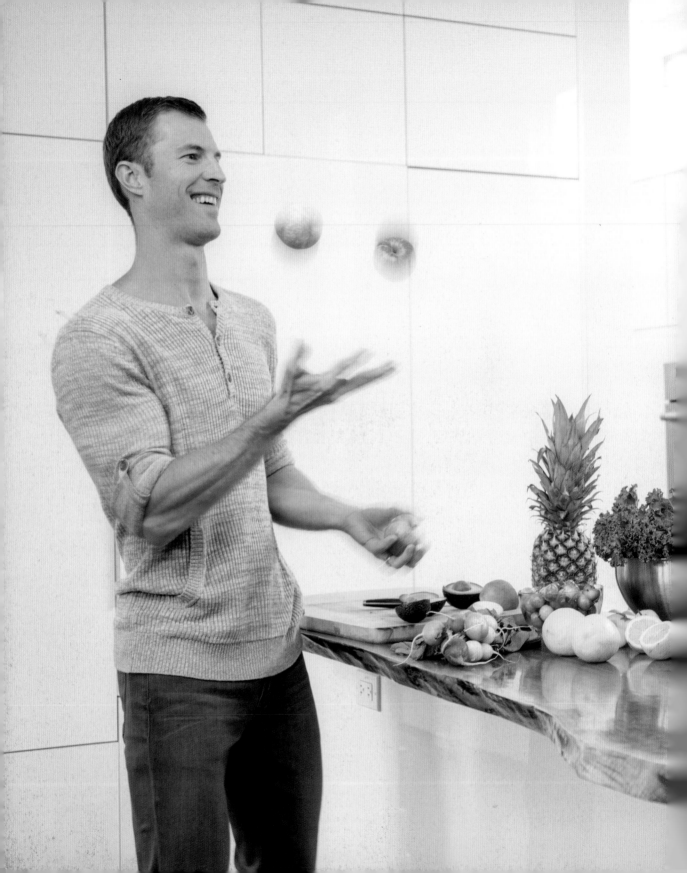

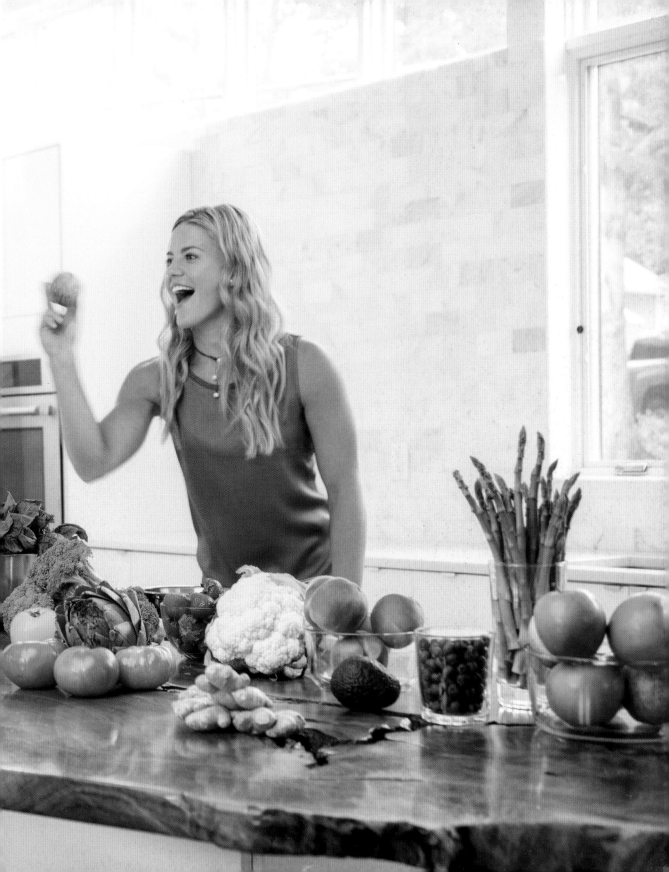

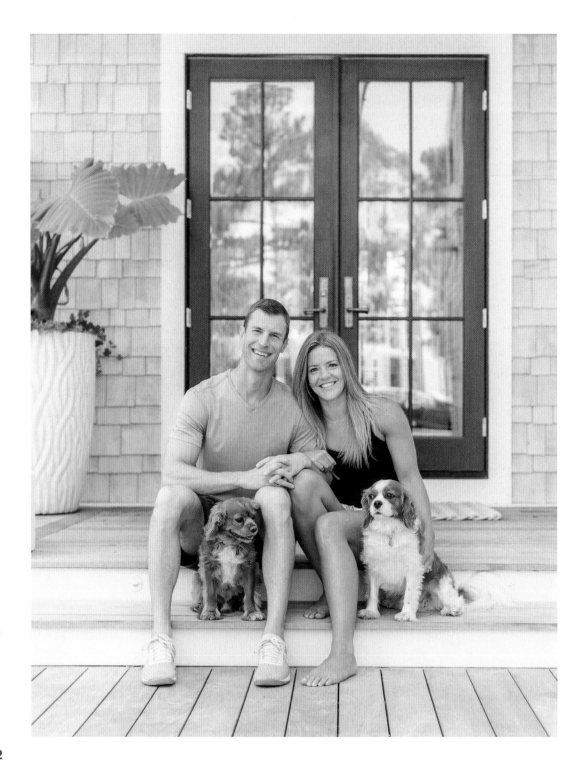

Acknowledgments

I want to thank the brilliant Ginny Graves for helping me create this book. Also, my sincere thanks to the entire Little, Brown Spark team, especially Tracy Behar and Peggy Freudenthal, for their fantastic insights, editing, and vision for what this book could be. I am grateful to my literary agent, Bonnie Solow, who is the best in the business and always goes above and beyond. I also want to express my heartfelt gratitude to Jordan Rubin, my closest friend and business partner, for inspiring me to write this book. And to my entire team at Ancient Nutrition: Thank you for all your hard work and sincere commitment to improving the health of our country and our world. Finally, my deepest appreciation to those of you who follow me on social media and visit my website—and who bought this book. Here's to you for investing in your well-being and taking your health to the next level!

Big Blessings!
Dr. Josh Axe

Index

Page number in *italics* indicate photographs or illustrations.